THE TRIATHLETE'S GUIDE TO

Mental Training

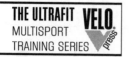

THE ULTRAFIT **VELO** MULTISPORT TRAINING SERIES press

Following the successful program of the Ultrafit coaches, these books will provide you with a specific map to build your strength and endurance in every facet of triathlon for a successful racing season.

Going Long: Training for Ironman-Distance Triathlons, Joe Friel and Gordon Byrn

The Triathlete's Guide to Bike Training, Lynda Wallenfels

The Triathlete's Guide to Half-Ironman Training, Tom Rodgers

The Triathlete's Guide to Mental Training, Jim Taylor and Terri Schneider

The Triathlete's Guide to Off-Season Training, Karen Buxton

The Triathlete's Guide to Run Training, Ken Mierke

The Triathlete's Guide to Swim Training, Stephen Tarpinian

Also from the Ultrafit Multisport Training Series:

Evolution Running DVD, featuring Ken Mierke from Endurance Films

You can find all of the Ultrafit titles at www.velopress.com.

Mental Training

Jim Taylor, Ph.D., and Terri Schneider

VELO press®

Boulder, Colorado

The Triathlete's Guide to Mental Training

Printed in the United States of America.
10 9 8 7 6 5 4 3 2 1

Distributed in the United States and Canada by Publishers Group West.

Library of Congress Cataloging-in-Publication Data
Taylor, Jim, 1958–
    The Triathlete's Guide to Mental Training / Jim Taylor and Terri Schneider.
        p. cm.
    Includes bibliographical references and index.
    ISBN 1-931382-70-0 (pbk : alk. paper)
        1. Triathlon—Psychological aspects. 2. Triathlon—Training.
    I. Schneider, Terri. II. Title.
    GV1060.73.T39 2005
    796.42'57—dc22

                                                          2005011109

VeloPress®
1830 North 55th Street
Boulder, Colorado 80301-2700 USA
303/440-0601 • Fax 303/444-6788 • E-mail velopress@insideinc.com

To purchase additional copies of this book or other VeloPress® books, call
800/234-8356 or visit us on the Web at velopress.com.

Cover design by Erin Johnson. Cover photo by Timothy Carlson.
Composition by Kate Hoffhine.

Contents

Foreword by Mark Allen

From my very first triathlon in June of 1982, I felt the profound effect one's mental attitude has on race performance. My sport background was age-group swimming, an endeavor where my results were mediocre at best. I never achieved a high level of success in the pool even though I was one of the toughest swimmers in the low-stress environment of a workout. In retrospect I can tell you with complete confidence that my lack of big results in big races was from my lack of mental training. If someone gained even a half-stroke lead over me in a swimming race, it was over. I could never come back once I was behind.

This wasn't so in my first triathlon I did on the beaches north of San Diego in Southern California. In that race I surprisingly started the run segment in fourth place, well ahead of any expectation I had going into my triathlon initiation. Within the first mile, however, another athlete ran by me like I was standing still. Immediately the swimmer tape began to roll right on cue, the one that told me I had been passed and there was nothing I could do about it.

But then something happened that laid the foundation for eventually winning the Ironman in Kona seven years later. It occurred to me that maybe, just maybe, getting passed was not the nail in the coffin. Just maybe if I relaxed and took the pass in stride, the dynamic of the race could turn back around. About a mile later it did indeed change. The runner who passed me stopped pulling away. A mile after that I was closing back in on him, and with less than two miles to go in the run, I passed him and moved back into fourth place. The three athletes who came in ahead of me represented the best the sport had to offer in the early 1980s. Finishing in first was Dave Scott. In second was Scott Molina, and in third was Scott Tinley. Among them over the course of their careers they amassed a total of nine Ironman world championship titles. On the surface, my result seemed both surprising and intriguing, solely because of who was ahead of me at the finish line. I was the next guy behind the best in the world.

The real success for me on that day was winning the mental race. It was the reason that I finished so high in the standings. I had changed the mental tape that had played so loudly for so many years. A window opened up for me that showed how much impact one's mind and heart has on the results at the finish line.

From that moment forward I began to explore every avenue possible to help develop my mental fitness. This ended up being the key element that enabled me to achieve some of the greatest successes in my career, most notably at the Ironman in Kona. Seven years after this first race, I was able to defeat the master of Kona, Dave Scott, in what has been called one of the greatest triathlon races of all time.

Dave Scott and I raced side by side the entire day. Then on the final uphill leading back into the town of Kona and the finish line I made a move that Dave could not answer. There had been no less than a thousand moments leading up to that decisive break in which I questioned whether or not I had what it took to beat the best in the sport. There were untold times when I wanted to just quit because the intensity of racing right next to such a strong competitor was more than I could have ever anticipated.

But every time, the answers needed to get me past each challenge came. Trust and faith in life itself, quieting my mind, surrendering to a race dynamic that had no resemblance to my pre-race visualization all played into the success I had on that day.

Without proper physical training I would not have had what it took to pull away from Dave. But what got me to the point where I was even next to him at the moment that counted was completely due to the attention I had given to working on my mental game in the years leading up to that decisive point in time.

You don't have to be a world-class athlete to reap the benefits of a good mental outlook. *The Triathlete's Guide to Mental Training* will show you this. It will also provide you with priceless tools to develop your own personal strength that comes from having the right mental focus. You will experience firsthand how valuable this is in creating the race performances that only come when mind and body are working together.

Even though the canvas of this book is painted in terms of swim, bike, and run, the tools you will find inside can help you find the right mental attitude in any area of your life. And it goes without saying that we can all benefit from adopting a positive outlook on life!

Best of luck with your training, racing, and life.

MARK ALLEN

SIX-TIME IRONMAN WORLD CHAMPION

Foreword by Michellie Jones

All athletes train hard. What makes some athletes champions and others not is their mental ability. I have seen so many athletes over the years who have the ability physically but never reach their full potential. Why? Because they never learned how to train their minds. When I am racing in a triathlon, it often comes down to not who has trained the hardest but who can handle the mental stress.

At the 1997 ITU World Triathlon Championships in Perth, Australia, I was in the lead group entering the transition from the bike to the run when one of the other competitors ran her bike right into me. I was knocked down and landed in her bladed spoke wheels. After struggling to get up, I quickly glanced down at my bare feet and couldn't see anything too badly wrong with me. I quickly put on my running shoes and caught up with the leaders. At about the two-mile mark of the run, I starting feeling weak. But I just kept telling myself I had done the training and I had to stay strong. At about four miles into the run, I started to lose a little ground to the leaders. My first thought was, "What is going on here?" Little did I know that I was leaving footprints of blood as I was running. With two miles to go, I was getting weaker and weaker, but I just willed myself to get through the next few minutes and hold on for third. I almost fainted when I crossed the finish line. Finally, I looked down and saw all the blood on my shoes. I ended up having four stitches in one foot and three in the other. Though I didn't win, I was as proud of my effort as much as either of my world titles because I could have given up, but I stayed positive and tough.

The Triathlete's Guide to Mental Training is a must-read for anyone who wants to overcome the physical and competitive challenges of triathlon. There are so many great insights and practical tools for triathletes to use in this book. And it is really easy to read. I wish I had read it early in my career. Even after competing for over 18 years, it reminded me of a few things I need to work on.

MICHELLIE JONES
TWO-TIME ITU WORLD CHAMPION

Acknowledgments

From Jim:

The Golden Gate Triathlon Club for allowing me to use its members as a sounding board and a source of valuable information and wonderful insights about the tri-life.

Duane Franks, Ironman triathlete, coach, and friend, for introducing me to the sport that has become a professional focus and a personal passion.

Terri Schneider, who brought passion and commitment to the book.

My father, Shel, and my late mother, Ceci, for instilling in me a lifelong passion for sport and psychology.

My wife, Sarah. Meeting at our first open-water swim in San Francisco's Aquatic Park on that cold and rainy day in March 2002 changed my life.

From Terri:

Dave Scott, Mike Pigg, Paul Huddle, Heather Fuhr, Victor Plata, Scott Tinley, Pete Kain, Mark Allen, and Michellie Jones for offering pieces of their unique lives within the sport of triathlon. Thanks for the sharing, the reminiscing, and the laughter.

Jim Taylor, who offered his wisdom and experience.

Heidi Vandegrift, for her patience while I took time away from our business for this project.

All the triathletes I have had the pleasure of coaching. Your efforts and passions are a constant inspiration.

The sport of triathlon. It's within this astounding sport that I initially grew and flourished as an athlete and as a woman and started to learn the beauty of pushing beyond limits.

My family for their lifelong and unconditional support of my endeavors, and friends for being solid sounding boards for this project; in particular, my mom, my sister Stephanie, Dave Liotta, Kevin Hume, Flo and Charlie Stover, Luanne Park, and David Terry.

Introduction

When you compete in a triathlon, you're competing in two races. The obvious race is the swim, bike, and run. The more significant race, though, is the race that occurs within your mind. Succeed in the mental race and you will succeed in the triathlon. Contrary to what many triathletes believe, at whatever level in which you're competing, the physical aspects of triathlon don't usually determine who is most successful. Triathletes who compete at the same level are very similar physically. Is Chris McCormack more fit than Craig Walton? Is Natasha Badmann stronger than Heather Fuhr? In both cases, the answer, most likely, is no, and this may be true for you and the triathletes you compete against. On any given day, what separates Peter Reid from Jergen Zack or Barbara Lindquist from Sheila Taormina? The answer lies in who succeeds in the mental race. Triathletes who are the most motivated to train, who have the greatest confidence in themselves, who race best under pressure, who stay focused on their race, who keep their emotions under control, and who can overcome the pain on race day will most often achieve their triathlon goals.

IMPORTANCE OF MENTAL PREPARATION

We often ask triathletes what aspect of the sport has the greatest impact on how they perform. Almost unanimously they say the mental side. We then ask how much time they devote to their mental preparation. Their answer most often is little or no time. Despite its obvious importance, the mental side of triathlon is often neglected, at least until a problem arises. You do physical conditioning to maximize your fitness and prevent injury. You practice your swim stroke to address technique flaws. You should approach your mental preparation in the same way.

We wrote *The Triathlete's Guide to Mental Training* to assist you in just this process, ensuring that mentally you're your best ally in your training and races. Within the book, we focus on the essentials of mental preparation and show you how to make your mind a valuable tool in your triathlon efforts. Just as an efficient and consistent training program offers you increased physical strength and stamina, the information within this book offers you the possibility of mental strength and resilience.

The Triathlete's Guide to Mental Training describes issues and concerns that are common to triathletes regardless of their ability or experience. The information, techniques, and exercises are designed to be easy to understand and apply directly to your training and race efforts. You will be able to use the techniques immediately to improve your training and race performances.

We wrote this book to benefit triathletes at all levels of the sport. Whether you're a "tri-newbie," a seasoned age grouper, or a top professional, or you compete in sprints, Olympic-distance, or Ironman races, the information and tools we provide can help you achieve your triathlon training and race goals.

> *The mental aspect is an area that many athletes can improve on. There are many aspects of sport psychology, the most important of which are confidence, motivation, concentration, and relaxation.*
>
> —Joe Friel, triathlon coach

The Triathlete's Guide to Mental Training has several goals: first, to provide clear and understandable information about succeeding in the mental race of triathlon; second, to offer simple and practical techniques that you can use to raise your performances to a new level; third, to enable you to perform your best consistently in your triathlon training and racing; and finally, to allow you to gain the greatest amount of satisfaction and joy possible from your involvement in the sport.

USING THE TRIATHLETE'S GUIDE TO MENTAL TRAINING

Given that there's a great deal of information in this guide, take your time absorbing each section. You'll most likely need to read some chapters several times. Just as it takes time to develop your physical and technical abilities, it will also take time to develop your mental capabilities, so be patient and commit yourself to your mental training the way you do to your physical and technical training.

The Triathlete's Guide to Mental Training has been organized around what we believe are the mental issues that most influence triathlon performance. This structure enables you to select the areas most relevant to your level of training and racing. It allows you to find out exactly what you need to know for where you are in your triathlon participation and development, and it describes in detail the information and skills you need to develop for the mental areas that are most important to you.

We suggest the following process in using *The Triathlete's Guide to Mental Training* to its greatest benefit. First, read the book all the way through. As you read, make note of specific topics that are currently important to you. After reading the entire book, identify the issues that are most pertinent to you and reread those sections to better familiarize yourself with them. Then, select two or three areas on which you want to focus. Experiment with different techniques to develop the areas you've chosen and select the ones you like best. Finally, implement those techniques in your training schedule.

Now, let's begin the exciting journey that culminates with you succeeding in the mental race and achieving your triathlon goals.

PART ONE

Building a Foundation for Triathlon Success

1

Introduction to Prime Triathlon

We would like to introduce you to several key concepts that will act as the foundation for *The Triathlete's Guide to Mental Training*. One of the most popular phrases used in sports is peak performance. It has become a common part of our vocabulary, used by athletes, coaches, and sport psychologists, as well as businesspeople and other high-level performers. Peak performance is typically defined as the highest level of performance a person can achieve and is considered to be the goal toward which all athletes should strive. When Jim came out of graduate school, peak performance was what he wanted the athletes with whom he worked to achieve.

But as Jim became more experienced as a psychologist and a writer, he began to appreciate the power of words and how vital it is that the words we use are specific to what we want to communicate. He saw several difficulties with the essence of peak performance. Triathletes can only maintain a peak for a very short time. Would you be satisfied if you performed well in one race and then did poorly in subsequent events? Also, once that peak is reached, there is only one way to go, and that is down.

So Jim searched for several years to find a phrase that accurately described what he wanted athletes to achieve. One day, while walking through the meat section of a grocery store, he saw a piece of beef with a sticker that read "Prime Cut." He knew he was on to something. He looked up "prime" in the dictionary and found it defined as "of the highest quality or value." Thus "Prime Performance" was born—a phrase highly descriptive of what he wanted athletes to achieve.

Prime Performance or, in this case, Prime Triathlon, is defined as "performing at a consistently high level under the most challenging conditions." There are two essential words in this definition. The first key word is "consistently." We want you to be able to perform at a high level day in and day out, week in and week out, month in and month out. Prime Performance is not about being "on" 100 percent of the time—that is impossible—but rather performing at a high level with only minimal ups and downs instead of the large swings in training and competitive performance that are so common among triathletes. The second key word is "challenging." It can be easy to have a good race under ideal conditions against an easy field in an unimportant race. What makes the great triathletes successful is their ability to perform their best under the worst possible conditions against a formidable field in the most important race of their lives. If you attain this level of performance, Prime Triathlon, you will not only be successful, but you will gain immense enjoyment and satisfaction from your efforts. Now that is a goal worth achieving!

> *When you're on, really recognize everything that feels like you're on. Be acutely aware emotionally, psychologically, physically how you feel. Then make it finite—what do your quads feel like right now? I'm running 5:30 pace and I'm really fluid, how do my calves feel, quads—so when I get in a race I would go back to that. You see yourself being fluid in your mind, and I'd see myself on the bike floating, like my foot is just floating through each motion. "It feels effortless now." Remember that.*
>
> —Dave Scott,
> six-time Ironman world champion

Where does Prime Triathlon come from? Though we'll be focusing on its mental contributors, the mind is only one piece of the puzzle. You also need to be at a high level of physical health, including being well conditioned, well rested, free from injury and illness, and eating a balanced diet. Your technical skills must be well learned and your tactics ingrained. If you're physically, technically, tactically, and mentally prepared, then you will have the ability to achieve Prime Triathlon.

Have you ever experienced Prime Triathlon? Do you know what it feels like to perform at that level? Let's describe some of the common experiences of Prime Triathlon. First, it is effortless—comfortable, easy, natural, and automatic. There's little thought; the body does what it knows how to do and there's no mental interference. You also experience sharpened senses; you see, hear, and feel everything more acutely. We've heard pros say that when they're experiencing Prime Triathlon, the distances seem shorter and the climbs feel less steep. You're totally absorbed in the experience and are focused entirely on the process. You have no distractions or unnecessary thoughts that interfere with your performance. You have boundless energy. Your endurance seems never-ending and fatigue is simply not an issue. Finally, you experience what we call Prime Integration. Everything is working together. The physical, technical, tactical, and mental aspects of the sport are integrated into one directed effort at achieving your goals and loving the triathlon experience.

PHILOSOPHY OF PRIME TRIATHLON

Before you can begin the process of developing Prime Triathlon, you want to create a foundation of beliefs about triathlon on which you can build your mental skills. This foundation involves your attitude in three areas: (1) your perspective on competition—what you think of it, how you feel about it, and how you approach it; (2) your view of yourself as a competitor—how you perform in training and races; and (3) your attitude toward success and failure—how you define success and failure and whether you know the essential roles that both success and failure play in becoming the best triathlete you can be. Clarifying your views in these three areas will make it easier to win the mental race and to achieve Prime Triathlon.

PERSPECTIVE ON TRIATHLON

Triathlon is important to you. You put a great deal of time and effort into your triathlon training and races. You give your best effort in every swim, bike, and run session. A difficult day of training or a poor race leaves you feeling disappointed. These feelings are natural because you care about triathlon. They motivate you to do better in the future.

There can be, however, a point at which you can lose perspective, and your feelings toward triathlon can hurt your training and race performances.

One of the most harmful words in triathlon is a simple three-letter word: T-O-O, too. You want to care about your triathlon participation, but you don't want to care *too* much. You want triathlon to be important to you, but you don't want it to be *too* important. You want to try to perform your best, but you don't want to try *too* hard.

In the "too zone," triathlon is no longer a positive aspect of your life— it is your life! Triathlon is no longer about having fun and achieving your goals. You invest your ego—how you feel about yourself as a person—in your training and competitive efforts. If training and races don't go well, you may dwell on these failings, feel bad about yourself, and become depressed and despondent. If you feel this way, it's important to step back and regain perspective. Reevaluate what triathlon means to you, the role it plays in your life, and how it affects your well-being and happiness. You may find that it plays too big of a role in your life. If triathlon defines how you feel about yourself, it will likely interfere with your achieving your triathlon goals and detract from the satisfaction you derive from the sport.

> ▼
>
> *I'm not psycho about winning or anything; I just try to do my best and enjoy the day, so every year I go to simply have a great time. I'm too old to go really deep, but I do enjoy competition and the goal of doing my best no matter what my age.*
>
> —Missy LeStrange, ten-time Ironman age-group champion

To perform your best and have fun, keep triathlon in perspective. Remember why you participate; it's fun, you enjoy the exercise, it's a great way to socialize, it's fulfilling to master a sport, and you enjoy the competition and achievements. The Prime Triathlon view of competition means that triathlon is a healthy and balanced part of your life that enhances you physically, mentally, socially, and spiritually. Have fun, give your best effort, enjoy the process of the sport, and you will perform better and attain your goals.

UPS AND DOWNS OF TRIATHLON

Another aspect of the Prime Triathlon perspective on competition is recognizing and accepting the ups and downs of the sport. In the history of triathlon, very few triathletes have had perfect or near-perfect seasons. Even the best triathletes have ebbs and flows within their seasons. The focus is not on whether you have ups and downs, but rather on the heights of the peaks and the depths of the valleys and how you respond to them. *The Triathlete's Guide to Mental Training* is devoted to assisting you in smoothing out the bumps in your season.

In a down period, it's easy to get down on yourself. You may feel disappointed and helpless to reverse this downward trend. You may want to give up. Stopping the descent and returning to a high level of performance is an essential skill for triathletes. Successful triathletes know how to stop their decline and regain a positive attitude, helpful emotions, and quality performance.

The first step to reversing your down period is to keep the ups and downs in perspective by knowing that they're a natural and expected part of the sport. This attitude takes the pressure off the down moments, minimizing frustration and disappointment. It enables you to stay positive and motivated. Most important, never give up. Stay focused on your triathlon goals. Look for the cause of your slump and find a solution. Maintaining this positive attitude toward the ups and downs of triathlon will help you keep the down periods short and help you return quickly to the highs.

> *I've learned how to deal with the ups and downs through years of experience. Being out there year in and year out, racing against young and old, short course and long, flat and hilly. Having raced in every condition imaginable. Heat, humidity, cold, wet, snow, I've seen it all and I've learned how to deal with it.*
> —Pete Kain, three-time ITU world age-group champion

TRIATHLON IS ABOUT LOVE

It's easy to lose sight of why you do triathlons. There are the races, competition, and attention. There are the cool bikes and other tri-gear. There are the fit and tanned bodies. Focusing on these external aspects of triathlon can cause you to lose sight of the deeper, more meaningful reasons why you participate. When external aspects of the sport become your focus, it's important to remind yourself what triathlon means to you.

If you think about it, triathlon is child's play. In a triathlon, you're doing what you used to love to do as a child. Every time you go for a swim, bike, or run, you have the opportunity to reconnect with the simplicity and purity of childhood. Remember the love you felt for those activities and the joy they brought you when you were young. It wasn't about being the best swimmer, pushing yourself in training, or having good race results, but rather the simple pleasure of splashing around the pool, speeding your bike down the street, or racing around your house on foot. What a wonderful gift that is. You can experience those same feelings as an adult triathlete. You can still just love to get out there and swim, bike, and run. You can love the triathlon community, which is full of vital and energetic people. The friendships you gain from triathlon can be just as enriching and fun. It can move, inspire, and help you grow as a person, enhancing all aspects of your life. Triathlon can provide you with meaning, satisfaction, and joy that can be unparalleled.

I just needed a shift in my racing mentality. It happened; it was a long process, but finally it did. It made me realize exactly why I'm doing this sport. It became a business for a while, and I just wasn't enjoying it anymore. All of a sudden I'm just doing it because I love it. All that downtime made me realize why I'm doing this.

—Peter Reid, three-time Ironman world champion

PRIME TRIATHLON FOR SUCCESS AND FAILURE

Your attitude toward success and failure also affects your involvement in triathlon. How you define success and failure will determine your ability to perform your best consistently and enjoy the sport. Too often, success and failure in our culture are defined narrowly; if you win, you succeed; if you don't, you fail. A wonderful aspect of triathlon is that, in any race, everyone can be a success. For some triathletes, adhering to their training program and getting to the start line is a success. For others, finishing a distance that they never imagined possible is a success. For still others, success might mean setting a personal best for the distance. And for the rare few, an age-group victory, a Kona slot, or an overall race win is a success. With this perspective in mind, we define success as giving your best effort, performing to the best of your ability, and enjoying the race experience. Because this definition of success is entirely within your control, you have the power to pursue and achieve success at will.

There are many myths and misconceptions that triathletes hold about success and failure. Many triathletes believe that the only way to succeed is to have always been successful; that successes rarely fail. But the reality is the most successful triathletes failed frequently and often monumentally on the path to success. Recall Peter Reid's near-career-ending failure in the 2001 Ironman® World Championships before his second-place finish in 2002 and his return in 2003 to win his third title. In fact, both successful and poor performances are essential to becoming a consistent success.

Poor performances in training and races provide you with information about your progress. They show you what you're doing well and, more importantly, what you need to improve on. Setbacks also show you what doesn't work, which helps you identify what works best. Poor performances also teach you how to positively respond to adversity, which is a common part of triathlon. Finally, setbacks teach you humility and an appreciation for what it takes to be successful. Because of the frequent and diverse challenges that triathlon throws at you and the frequent and oftentimes painful lessons it teaches, you develop a healthy respect for the

> *I know it's a bit of a cliché—"Do the best you can"—but what more can you do? If you're strong upstairs, then you'll race well. There's not much more you can do than concentrate on your own day and just get out there and give it a go.*
>
> —Spencer Smith, three-time ITU world champion

sport as well as for your ability to learn those lessons. Rather than becoming disheartened by poor performances, focus on how they will help you become a better triathlete.

Of course, too much failure can be discouraging. You need to experience success to continue to improve as a triathlete. Success builds confidence and reinforces your belief that you can perform well and meet the challenges of competition. There are, however, problems with being successful too often. Success can breed complacency, because if you succeed all of the time, there's little motivation to improve. Sooner or later though, as you move up the competitive ladder, you'll come up against others who are just as good as or better than you, and since you haven't put in the time and effort to improve, you won't be successful against them. Also, always succeeding may not allow you to recognize areas in need of improvement. If you learn the valuable lessons from both success and failure, you'll gain the perspective that will allow you to achieve Prime Triathlon.

PRIME TRIATHLETE

Looking back at the great competitors in triathlon over the years from Dave Scott and Karen Smyers to Mike Pigg and Paula Newby-Fraser to Chris McCormack and Michellie Jones, you see common qualities that make them champions. Each has unique abilities, styles, and personalities, but all share several essential characteristics.

While competing, all of these triathletes were in top physical condition and technically proficient. But there are many triathletes who have these same qualities who don't achieve greatness. Performing your best requires that you have all of the qualities you would expect a great triathlete to possess: physically well conditioned, excellent technique, and sound tactics. These attributes will only make you a good triathlete. Becoming a prime triathlete, like those just mentioned, requires something more.

There's a considerable difference between performing well in training, in races, and in the most important race of the year. This difference is what separates most triathletes from prime triathletes. You must first get into top physical condition, develop sound technical skills, and understand the tactical aspects of the sport. The final challenge is learning what it takes to succeed in the mental race and to evolve from a triathlete to a prime triathlete.

Prime triathletes generally train well, but they may not, for example, be at the front of the long rides or lead the pack during track workouts. They may have poor performances in less important races. But what separates prime triathletes from others is how they respond to adversity and pressure. In important races against topflight fields under difficult conditions, their performances rise to a new level. Everything that turns negative for most triathletes shifts positively for prime triathletes, and this ability to rise to the occasion propels them to the top.

At the heart of all prime triathletes is an unwavering determination to be the best. They are driven to constantly improve. They have great passion for hard work. They spend hours each day training to increase their performance. They embrace the repetition of training, and they're willing to suffer to succeed. Their love of the sport precedes their love of competing and winning.

Prime triathletes have a deep and enduring belief in themselves. They have the confidence to push their limits, to endure discomfort in training and races, and to never give up. This belief enables them to be inspired by defeat and allows them to keep faith in their ability even when faced with adversity. Difficult conditions and tough competition are exciting challenges and opportunities to showcase their skills.

Prime triathletes are able to raise their performances in order to succeed. They thrive on the pressure of significant events, like the Olympics, the ITU World Championships, and Hawaii Ironman®. They've developed the ability to stay calm and focused with a championship on the line. Most fundamentally, prime triathletes perform their best in the most important races of their lives.

Becoming a prime triathlete requires that you maximize every aspect of your athletic ability. It starts at the physical level. An optimal level of fitness results from being committed to a quality training program aimed at achieving your triathlon goals. Though not often thought of as a technical sport by laypeople, those in the know realize that each of the three disciplines of triathlon has its own technical demands that must be mastered to perform at a high level. You need to develop ingrained and automatic technique that withstands fatigue and pain. You must also have tactical skills and strategy for the type of course, weather conditions, and distance of the race in which you compete. These efforts, however, will only take you part of the way down the road to becoming a prime triathlete.

One of the noble lessons from the sport of triathlon is that we can shape ourselves and our surroundings mentally, physically, and emotionally. . . . Triathletes are indeed the "new Jedi order" of highly trained mental and physical giants.

—Mitch Thrower, triathlon journalist

Motivation is the key to putting in the time and effort necessary to be physically, technically, tactically, and mentally prepared. You need to develop confidence that you can perform well in the most important race of your life under the most demanding conditions. You must train yourself to seek out and thrive on adversity and have the ability to stay calm and focused when the race is on the line. You need the ability to use your emotions to your advantage so that they help you perform well. Finally, mastering the pain that you will experience in training and races will enable you to endure the physical challenges you will face as you pursue your goals.

But you don't have to be a pro triathlete, or even a top age grouper, to be a prime triathlete. Every triathlete can become one. You'll notice that none of the attributes we just described have anything to do with natural ability or winning. Every one of those qualities can be learned by any triathlete to achieve their personal best. *The Triathlete's Guide to Mental Training* is devoted to helping you become a prime triathlete, to be thoroughly prepared for every competition, physically, technically, tactically, and mentally ready to perform your best.

MIND IN CHARGE

Experienced triathletes will tell you that once you've done your training, a triathlon is a greater challenge mentally than it is physically. Late in the race when your body starts to break down, your mind may struggle with remaining positive and motivated. Your body may scream at you, "I hate this! I'm going to stop now!" If your mind agrees with your body and responds, "You're right. This hurts too much. I can't go on," you'll slow down or stop, and you won't achieve your goals.

> *In the beginning it's hard to understand that the race is not against others but against that little voice in your head that tells you when to quit.*
> —Charles Brenke,
> age-group triathlete

The best chance you have to tap into that final reserve of energy that will get you to the finish line is for your mind to encourage, cajole, and persuade your body to keep going in the face of fatigue and pain. If you can say, "Keep at it. This is what I've worked so hard for. I will not give up," then your body will listen—however reluctantly—and you will cross the finish line having succeeded against the course, the clock, and, most importantly, yourself.

PRIME TRIATHLON SKILLS ARE SKILLS

Some triathletes have misconceptions about the mental side of sport. They may believe that mental abilities are inborn—we either have them or we don't. But mental abilities are skills, just like technical skills, that can be developed. You can approach mental skills the same way that you approach physical and technical parts of triathlon. If you consistently work on them, your mental skills will improve and your overall performance rise.

PRIME TRIATHLON PYRAMID

The goal of *The Triathlete's Guide to Mental Training*, helping you experience the feeling and performance of Prime Triathlon, is accomplished by ascending the Prime Triathlon pyramid, which is comprised of six mental factors that most influence triathlon performance: motivation, confidence, intensity, focus, emotions, and pain. These six mental factors are ordered such that each area builds on the previous ones, leading to Prime Triathlon (see Figure 1.1).

At the base of the Prime Triathlon pyramid lies *motivation*, which is essential for maintaining the desire and determination to train. Prime motivation ensures that you put in the necessary time and effort to be totally prepared to perform your best. From motivation to prepare comes *confidence* in your physical, technical, tactical, and mental capabilities, and in your ability to achieve your goals. Prime confidence gives you the desire to compete and a core belief that you can perform well. From confidence comes the ability to manage your *intensity* and respond positively to the demands and pressures of competition. Prime intensity enables you to maintain your ideal

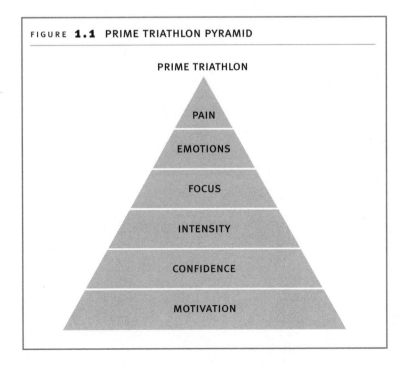

FIGURE **1.1** PRIME TRIATHLON PYRAMID

PRIME TRIATHLON

PAIN

EMOTIONS

FOCUS

INTENSITY

CONFIDENCE

MOTIVATION

Many triathletes still don't do any mental training, and among those who do, most do it only in the final hours or days before big races. Mental training needs to happen year-round.

—Dave Scott

intensity throughout training and races. From intensity comes the ability to *focus* properly during your triathlon efforts. Prime focus lets you stay focused and avoid distractions. From motivation, confidence, intensity, and focus comes the ability to master your *emotions*. Prime emotions ensure that your emotions become a beneficial tool while training and competing. Finally, these five mental factors give you the skills necessary to overcome the *pain* that is an unavoidable part of triathlon training and racing. Having ascended the Prime Triathlon pyramid, you will have the tools to achieve Prime Triathlon.

TRIATHLETE SPOTLIGHT: DEBBIE

Debbie, at age 29, was new to triathlon, but already showed considerable promise. A former NCAA Division I runner, she quickly picked up swimming and cycling and emerged as a top age grouper in her first three years in the sport. With a full-time job and a low-key attitude toward triathlon—her training wasn't organized or intensive—she was having fun and getting great results. After two Ironman races, in which she finished reasonably high in her age group, she had a breakthrough Ironman performance in which she finished sixth overall. With this result, she decided to quit her job and turn pro.

She hired a coach and established a highly structured training program. Her triathlon life became her entire life and revolved around training, eating, and recovery every day. She lost touch with her nontriathlon friends and gave up several hobbies that she had enjoyed previously. Despite her commitment and efforts, Debbie had a terrible triathlon season. She found training a chore, monotonous and boring. Before races, she was so nervous, she thought she was going to be ill. Her races were a struggle and her results suffered. She seemed to be going backward. Following a string of poor races, she was disconsolate; frustrated, angry, and depressed. It took her a week and considerable coaxing from her coach and family to get her back to training. This pattern continued all year until she was just glad to have the season over with.

Having run out of money and realizing that a pro career wasn't in the cards, Debbie decided to return to school and just do triathlons for fun. She cut back on her training, doing just what she felt, reconnected with her friends, and got back into her hobbies. At her first race, she noticed that she wasn't even a bit nervous, had a fun time during the race, and, much to her surprise, won her age group (and beat several pros). Her successes—and her enjoyment—continued throughout the season and she has continued those successes and joy in triathlon ever since.

C H A P T E R

2 Prime Triathlon Profiling

The first step toward achieving Prime Triathlon is to gain a better understanding of yourself as a triathlete. Self-understanding is important in showing you your strengths and weaknesses and enabling you to see how you react in certain situations. This self-understanding results in faster progress. Becoming the best triathlete you can is complex. You have enormous time constraints with school, work, family, social life, and other activities. Gaining an understanding of yourself will enable you to be efficient and focused in your triathlon efforts.

In developing greater self-understanding, you need to recognize your strengths and weaknesses. Triathletes enjoy focusing on their strengths, but often have difficulty seeing or admitting their weaknesses. Some triathletes also think that they're as good as their greatest strengths. For example, a former collegiate runner who now competes in triathlon believes that his running endurance and speed will enable him to achieve his goals. The truth is, however, that triathletes are only as good as their most significant weakness. If the former runner lacks the power necessary to have a fast and efficient ride, any advantage he may have after T2 could be neutralized. Recognizing your weaknesses will foster their development and enhance your strengths. If, like the example above, cycling is your weakness and running your strength, you can optimize your running by increasing your cycling fitness. The less fatigued you are coming off the bike, the fresher your run will be.

Think of triathlon strengths and weaknesses as a mathematical equation (see Prime Profile Formula below). If a triathlete is an excellent swimmer (10), but she is a weak cyclist (2), and a mediocre runner (6), her overall performance would be low (10 + 2 + 6 = 18). If she worked on and improved her cycling (5) and running (8), then her overall performance would rise significantly (10 + 5 + 8 = 23). The more you improve your weaknesses, the greater the gains you can make in your overall performance.

PRIME PROFILE FORMULA

STRENGTHS + WEAKNESSES = OVERALL TRIATHLON PERFORMANCE

WHY PRIME TRIATHLON PROFILING?

You may find it challenging to grasp the mental aspects of triathlon because they're intangible and not easily measured. To learn about your physical strengths and weaknesses, you can go through a physical testing program that provides objective data about your physical condition; for example, you may have your VO_2max tested. Similarly, a video analysis or coach's assessment can objectify technical capabilities. Yet there are no direct ways to measure your mental strengths and weaknesses. You can, however, measure your "mental muscles" indirectly through the use of pencil-and-paper inventories. Prime Triathlon profiling has been developed for this exact purpose (see page 21). You can think of Prime Triathlon profiling as physical testing for the mind. It makes mental issues related to triathlon more concrete. Prime Triathlon profiling increases your self-understanding so you can take active steps to maintain your strengths and improve your weaknesses.

It's important for you to have an open mind with Prime Triathlon profiling. Consider the information in a positive and constructive way. When weaknesses are identified, it doesn't mean that you're incapable of performing well. It may be that you haven't had to use these skills at your current level or you've been able to hide them with your strengths. Knowing your strengths can give you confidence in your ability to meet the challenges of triathlon. Knowing your weaknesses gives you a starting point for minimizing your limitations and turning them into strengths.

COMPLETING THE PRIME TRIATHLON PROFILE

The Prime Triathlon profile is comprised of twelve mental, emotional, and competitive factors that influence triathlon performance. To complete the Prime Triathlon profile (see page 21), read the description of each factor below and rate yourself on a one-to-ten scale by drawing a line at that level and shading in the area toward the center of the profile.

- **Self-awareness** involves how well you know your mental strengths and weaknesses. Do you have an understanding of what helps and hurts you mentally? (1-don't know self; 10-know self well)
- **Motivation** refers to how determined you are to train and compete to achieve your triathlon goals. Motivation affects all aspects of your preparation, including your desire to put time and energy into physical conditioning, technical and tactical development, and mental preparation. Do you work consistently on all aspects of triathlon or do you try less hard or give up when you get tired, bored, or frustrated? (1-not at all motivated; 10-very motivated)
- **Confidence** relates to how strongly you believe in your ability to achieve your goals. It is reflected in how positive or negative your self-talk is in training and during races. Confidence includes how well you're able to maintain your confidence in races, especially when faced with challenging conditions. Do you stay confident and positive or do you lose confidence and become negative in difficult conditions and when you're not performing well? (1-very negative; 10-very positive)
- **Intensity** determines whether your physical state helps or hurts you in races. Are you able to stay calm and relaxed or are you too anxious before and during races? (1-anxious; 10-relaxed)
- **Focus** is concerned with how well you're able to keep your mind on performing your best during races. It involves avoiding distractions and staying focused. Are you able to stay focused on what you need to in order to perform well or do you become distracted by things that hurt your performances? (1-distracted; 10-focused)
- **Emotions** involve how well you're able to control your emotions before and during a race. In important races under difficult conditions or when you're not performing well, do you stay

excited and inspired or do you get frustrated, angry, or depressed? Do your emotions help or hurt you in races? (1-bad emotions, hurt; 10-good emotions, help)

- **Pain** refers to the amount of physical discomfort you experience in training and races and how you respond to it. Does the pain you feel interfere with your giving your best effort in training and races? Are you able to effectively master the pain you experience? (1-severe, can't master; 10-manageable, can master)

- **Consistency** relates to how well you're able to maintain your level of performance during a race. Does your level of performance stay at a consistently high level or does it go up and down frequently in races? (1-very inconsistent; 10-very consistent)

- **Quality** refers to how well you're able to maintain the highest-quality training with clear goals and purpose and ideal intensity and focus. Are your workouts of the highest quality or does their quality vary significantly? (1-poor quality; 10-high quality)

- **Adversity** is concerned with your ability to respond positively to adverse conditions and obstacles you're faced with in training and races. For example, how do you react when the conditions are cold and windy or when you get a flat or a cramp? (1-respond poorly; 10-respond well)

- **Role** involves whether triathlon plays a healthy or unhealthy role in your life. Does triathlon have a balanced place in your life and does it bring you satisfaction and joy or has it taken over your life and does it have more costs than benefits? (1-unhealthy; 10-healthy)

- **Prime Triathlon** refers to how often you achieve your highest level of training and race performance. Are you able to achieve Prime Triathlon regularly or is it a rare occurrence? (1-never; 10-often)

USING YOUR PRIME TRIATHLON PROFILE

Having completed the Prime Triathlon profile, you now have a clear picture of what you believe to be your mental strengths and weaknesses in triathlon. Typically, a score below a 7 indicates an area on which you need to focus. Place a √ next to each factor on which you scored less than a 7. You'll want to consider working on these factors in your mental training program.

From those checked factors, select three to focus on in the immediate future. It's most efficient to focus on a few, strengthen them, and then

PRIME TRIATHLON PROFILE

Directions: Twelve mental factors that influence triathlon performance are identified in the profile below. Using the definitions provided above, rate yourself on a 1–10 scale for each factor by drawing a line at that level and shading in the area toward the center of the profile. A score below a 7 indicates an area in need of improvement.

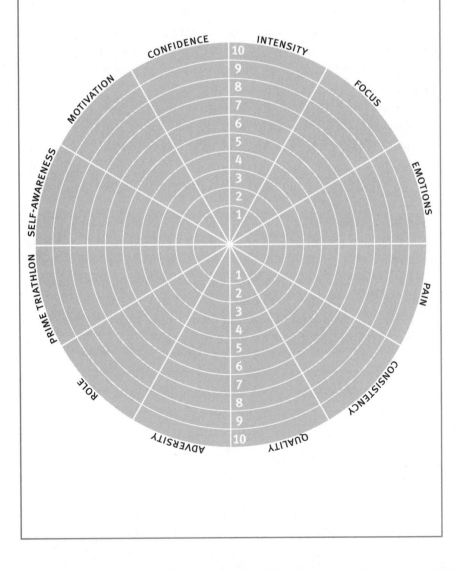

move on to the others. If you have more than three factors on which you need to work, which ones should you choose? The decision is based on several concerns. First, look at the factors that are most important for your development. For example, your ability to handle pain may be your biggest obstacle to achieving your goals, so this factor should have a high priority in your mental training. Second, some weaknesses are symptoms of other weaknesses. By dealing with one factor, another one may be relieved without having to work on it directly. For example, you may not handle adversity well because you lack confidence. By building your confidence, you also improve your ability to overcome adversity. Third, balance your immediate training and competitive needs with your long-term development. If you have an important race to prepare for and your lack of focus and intensity are holding you back, decide to improve those two mental areas immediately, even though working on your motivation and confidence may be more important in the future.

Using the Prime Triathlon priority form on page 23, indicate the three mental factors you want to focus on in the near future. After reading *The Triathlete's Guide to Mental Training*, return to the relevant chapters to learn about techniques and exercises that will help you strengthen the areas you've selected. Use the goal-setting program described in Chapter 9 to work on those areas.

You can also use Prime Triathlon profiling to measure progress in your training. Once a month, complete the profile and compare it with your past profiles. You should see improvement in the areas on which you've worked. If you have a coach or training partners, ask them to complete the profile based on their perceptions of you and any positive changes they've seen in those areas. When your ratings move above 7, select other factors to work on and follow the same procedure.

PRIME TRIATHLON PRIORITY FORM

Directions: In the space below, indicate three areas that you have identified in your Prime Triathlon profile on which you would like to focus. As these areas improve and new areas need work, complete this form again to specify the new priorities.

1.

2.

3.

TRIATHLETE SPOTLIGHT: SEAN

Sean, a 42-year-old, had been doing triathlons for eight years. He enjoys the sport, but was frustrated that he never seemed to race as well as he trained. He gave his best effort in training, was in good shape, and his goals seemed realistic, but his race performances were always disappointing. A voracious consumer of triathlon information, he was confident that his training program was sound and that he had no glaring technical weaknesses. After reading a sport psychology article in one of the triathlon magazines, he realized that his problems might be mental.

A self-proclaimed nonintrospective person, before the 2003 season, Sean began to explore the mental side of triathlon and was surprised at how little he had even thought, much less done, anything about it. He took the Prime Triathlon profile and began to see a pattern emerge in what was holding him back. He first realized that he didn't have much confidence in really pushing himself during a race. Thinking back to past races, he would think about picking up his pace, but didn't because he was afraid of bonking, even though he'd swum, biked, or run at the faster pace in training. He also realized that he didn't focus that well during races. Again thinking back to past races, he recognized that during most of the runs, he would find someone to talk to and, as a result, would slow his pace.

Sean applied this newfound self-awareness to his training and races that season. He worked on being positive and trusting his fitness as he raced more aggressively. He also consciously chose not to speak to other competitors during the run and focused on his pace. To his pleasant surprise, his race times improved noticeably over the previous year, his results got better, and he was having more fun than in any previous season.

PART TWO

Prime Triathlon Pyramid

CHAPTER

3 Motivation

M otivation lies at the base of the Prime Triathlon pyramid. It's the foundation on which everything you do in triathlon is built. Your motivation determines the priority you place on triathlon in your life, the amount of time you put into your training, how much mental preparation you do, and how much you push yourself in training and races. Without your desire and determination to train and compete, all of the other mental factors—confidence, intensity, focus, emotions, and pain—as well as the physical and technical elements of triathlon, are meaningless.

Motivation, simply defined, is the ability to initiate and persist at a task. To achieve your triathlon goals, you must be motivated to begin the process of developing as a triathlete. Your motivation will determine your effort in your training and races. Motivation in triathlon is imperative because you must be willing to maintain your efforts in the face of fatigue, boredom, pain, and other distractions. Motivation will determine the role that triathlon plays in your life and the choices you make around the sport. It will affect every aspect of your performance: physical conditioning, technical and tactical training, mental preparation, and general lifestyle, including sleep, diet, school or work, and relationships.

Motivation is the only contributor to your triathlon performance over which you have control. The Triathlon Performance Formula (see page 28) helps explain this notion. There are three aspects of triathlon that affect how well you perform. Your physical ability influences your performance, but though it can change somewhat over time with training, you are limited by your genetic makeup (such as body type, muscle composition, body fat content, and cardiovascular efficiency). The difficulty of the race, the competitiveness of the field, and the course and weather conditions affect how well you perform, but you have no control over these factors. Motivation will directly influence your development and the level of performance you ultimately achieve. If you're highly motivated to train, you'll put in the time and effort necessary to improve your conditioning, and your technical, tactical, and mental skills. Motivation will also affect your race performances. Your motivation will determine how you react to fatigue, pain, setbacks, and adversity.

> *I guess you can get muscle biopsies and that crap, but desire will always be the most important thing.*
> —Jimmy Riccitello, former pro triathlete

TRIATHLON PERFORMANCE FORMULA

ABILITY – DIFFICULTY OF COMPETITION + MOTIVATION = PERFORMANCE

WHY DO YOU DO TRIATHLONS?

To maximize your motivation, you need to understand why you do triathlons. Internal motivators can include having a great passion for the sport, enjoying the level of fitness that is gained, experiencing the "tri-high," overcoming the many challenges of triathlon, and embracing the meaning, satisfaction, and joy that the sport can provide. External motivators might be respect and attention from others, the deep friendships that can develop, and appreciating being outdoors.

Ask yourself why you do triathlons and what you gain from the sport. Knowing your motivations can help you create a "tri-life" that best satisfies your needs, maximizes your enjoyment, and ensures that you achieve your triathlon goals. For example, if you love to train, but don't enjoy racing that much, you might have an intense training program that focuses on only a few races a year. If you enjoy the people most, you might join a triathlon club and do masters swim sessions, group rides, and evening club track workouts.

If your motivation to participate in triathlons is to compete and perform your best, two questions you should ask yourself are, "How motivated am

I?" and "Am I as motivated as I need to be to achieve my triathlon goals?" Goals will not be fulfilled if you're not motivated to devote the time and energy to fulfill them. It's important that your motivation is consistent with your goals. Are you willing to do what is necessary to reach your goals? If not, then you have two choices: increase your motivation to attain your goals or lower your goals to a level you can achieve.

Motivation is also essential in your training. Motivation is the force that impels you to get out of bed in the morning to train or pushes you to work out after a long day of work. It determines the nature of your training and the frequency, volume, and intensity you have in your training. Motivation will keep you going when you're tired, bored, stressed, struggling, doing poorly, or not having fun.

▼

I know what hard work means and what it takes to excel. . . . Getting to the Olympics has always been a dream, but now it has become my number one goal. All I have to do is look at the Olympic rings. I am ready to go for almost every workout.

—Andy Potts,
2004 U.S. Olympic Triathlon Team

Obstacles to Motivation

Despite your best efforts to stay motivated and committed to triathlon, there are many obstacles that can arise that can prevent you from fully expressing the desire and determination you have to achieve your goals. There are many factors in your life that can inhibit your motivation. The chances are you have a busy life in which triathlon is only one part. Life stress from career or school, family and friends, and other commitments may cause your motivation to lag or disappear at times. Other causes of low motivation include overtraining, illness, injury, monotony, and loss of life balance.

SIGNS OF LOW MOTIVATION

There are some common signs of low motivation. A lack of desire to train as much as you have time to is one clear symptom. Less than 100-percent effort in training is another warning sign of low motivation. When you train, do you work as hard as necessary? Do you complete all aspects of your daily training program? Skipping or shortening training sessions or finding excuses to not work out are also common signs for triathletes with low motivation. If you're not motivated, it's easy to leave out or reduce parts of your training, particularly when it isn't enjoyable or is particularly difficult.

Another indication of low motivation is that you're simply not enjoying the sport. It's not likely that you're being forced to do triathlons. Ideally, you do them because you have fun and you gain a great deal from the sport. If training and races become a consistent chore, make some changes so you get the fun back in your tri-life and reconnect with your motivation to participate.

When I am having trouble motivating myself to train, I try and figure out why I am feeling that way.... It is essential to get to the root of the problem and to make the changes at a very fundamental level.

—Heather Fuhr,
1997 Ironman world champion

If you exhibit any of these signs of low motivation, it will be difficult to achieve your goals. If you're not as motivated as you want to be, do two things: first, ask yourself why you're not giving your best effort in training, and second, take active steps to increase your motivation in triathlon.

PRIME MOTIVATION

Prime motivation involves putting in as much time, effort, energy, and focus as you need to achieve your triathlon goals. It means training with sufficient frequency, volume, and intensity to get the most benefits from your involvement in triathlon, which can mean improvement, results, socializing, or fun. Whatever your main motivation is, prime motivation ensures that your motivation is satisfied.

Three Ds of Motivation

Prime motivation is based on what we call the three Ds (see page 31). The first D stands for *direction*. Before you can achieve prime motivation, you should first consider the different directions you can move in triathlon. You have three choices: stop participating completely, continue at your current level, or adjust your efforts up or down, depending on what you're striving to accomplish in the sport.

The second D represents *decision*. With these three choices of direction, select one direction in which to move. None of these directions is necessarily better or worse; they're simply your options. Your choice will dictate the amount of time and effort you put into triathlon and how good a triathlete you will ultimately become.

The third D stands for *dedication*. Once you've made your decision, dedicate yourself to it. Whatever decision you have made, commit yourself wholeheartedly to that course to achieve your goals. If your decision is to become the best triathlete you can be, then this last step, dedication, is absolutely critical to whether you realize that goal. Your decision to be your best and your dedication to triathlon must be a top priority. Only by being completely dedicated to your direction and decision will you ensure that you have prime motivation.

THREE Ds

DIRECTION → DECISION → DEDICATION → MOTIVATION

DEVELOPING MOTIVATION

You now have a better understanding of motivation and how it affects your triathlon efforts. If you're not as motivated as you'd like to be, you can change. We have provided below a variety of strategies you can use to improve your motivation.

Focus on your long-term goals. Though it's important to generate focused effort in triathlon, not all of that time and effort is enjoyable. We call this "the grind," which involves having to put hours upon hours of time and energy into training, often beyond the point of fun and excitement. During the grind, stay focused on your long-term goals and the result from committed effort—increased fitness, improved skills, and better performance—rather than on fatigue, pain, and boredom. Imagine what you want to accomplish. Remind yourself that the only way to reach your goals is to go through the grind. Generate the feelings of fulfillment and pride that you'll experience when you reach your goals. This technique will distract you from the unpleasantness of the grind, keep you focused on what you want to achieve, and generate positive thoughts and emotions that will help you through the grind.

Establish a support system. The people with whom you surround yourself have a significant impact on all aspects of your life. They affect what you think, how you feel, and how you act. These people also influence your motivation in triathlon. If you're around people who value and support your triathlon participation, you'll have an easier time staying motivated.

To constantly bolster your motivation, establish a support system that appreciates and encourages your triathlon efforts. This positive support system can include your immediate family, friends, and coworkers. Also, build a larger support system that fosters your motivation. Membership and participation in a local triathlon club can expose you to other like-minded people, group training experiences, educational opportunities to learn more about triathlon, and new friendships based on common interests and goals. A coach can motivate you by providing a wealth of valuable information about triathlon, ensuring that you train and race in a way that maximizes your progress.

When I am having a hard time motivating, I find a group to train with. I used to train by myself a lot when I was younger; back then there weren't too many groups to train with. Now I use the group rides, masters swims, and group track workouts to motivate me to get out there when I need a little extra push. Works every time.

—Pete Kain

It's difficult to be consistently motivated if you train alone. There are some days when you don't feel like getting out there and putting in the miles. And no matter how much you push yourself alone, you'll work that much harder if you have someone pushing you. Find a training partner who can help keep you motivated. Commitment to a training partner can motivate you to get out of bed at 5:00 A.M. for a masters swim or drag you to the track after work when you're tired. The best training partner is someone at about your level of ability who has similar goals. You may swim, bike, and run at the same pace and you may be training for the same distance race. You can work together and motivate each other to accomplish your goals. Your training is a shared commitment and responsibility that you must uphold for yourself and your training partner. When you're motivated, you not only help yourself, you also help your training partner. Having someone rely on you and having someone to depend on creates a collective motivation that is greater than the motivations of each individual.

Set goals. There are few experiences more rewarding and motivating than setting a goal, putting effort toward the goal, and reaching the goal.

The sense of achievement and validation of the effort inspires and motivates you to strive higher. It's valuable to establish clear goals of what you want to accomplish in triathlon and how you will achieve those goals. Seeing that your efforts lead to progress and results should motivate you further to pursue triathlon goals (Chapter 9 will show you how to create an organized goal-setting program).

Recognize your accomplishments. Recognizing your training efforts and accomplishments, and imagining how they benefit your triathlon progress, offers you a great opportunity to bolster your motivation. After every workout, stop and take stock of what you've done. Review the specifics of your training session. For example, go over the 3,000 yards of drills and intervals you just finished in the pool, the 2,500 feet of vertical you climbed on your bike, or the 4 x 800 repeats you just did on the track. Remind yourself of your effort and discomfort, all in the name of greater strength, speed, and stamina. Look forward and think about how that effort will help you achieve your triathlon goals. Finally, give yourself a pat on the back and allow yourself to feel the satisfaction and pride of a job well done.

Vary your workouts. Endurance sports can get monotonous and boring sometimes. Because of the importance of time-intensive repetition, it's valuable to boost motivation by varying your workouts. One reason many people take up triathlon is to engage in three different disciplines regularly. Too much of the same workout can suck the motivation right out of you. Overused workouts may drag down your motivation and decrease your intensity and focus, thus reducing their quality and the benefits and enjoyment you gain from them.

Having trouble motivating may also be a need to change things up a bit—to make the training more exciting with different workouts or different people to train with.

—Heather Fuhr

A way to stay motivated is to keep your workouts fresh by varying them frequently. You can alter your training by changing specific workouts, settings, or people. This change will prevent you from falling into a rut and just "going through the motions." New and creative workouts are motivating because they keep you interested and excited about your training. Varied workouts aid you in maintaining focus and intensity by requiring you to pay attention to the new routines and sustain the energy needed to perform them properly. The result is consistent, high-quality training that you enjoy.

Focus on your greatest competitor. Some triathletes are motivated by a goal of beating a fellow competitor. Because you don't have control over others' efforts, this external motivator may not be ideal. But for some, focusing on their greatest competitor can provide the impetus to work hard. If you feel this approach can work for you, identify your biggest competitor and put his or her name or photo where you can see it every day. Ask yourself, "Am I working as hard as him/her?" By maintaining your best effort, you have a chance to overcome your greatest competitor and achieve your goals.

> She [Erin Baker] became the motivating factor for me. She was the single factor that pushed me to a higher level at that time. I always felt that she was a better, more gifted athlete than I am. I always felt like I was the underdog. She threw her words around to mess you up mentally. As I got older, I used that as my motivating force.
> —Paula Newby-Fraser, eight-time Ironman world champion

Use motivational cues. A large part of staying motivated involves generating positive emotions associated with your efforts and goals. Feelings of pride and inspiration can bolster motivation during training and races. A way to create motivating emotions is with motivational cues, such as inspirational phrases and photographs. If you come across a quote or a picture that moves you, place it where you can see it regularly, such as in your bedroom, on your refrigerator door, or in your locker. Look at it periodically and allow yourself to experience the emotions it generates. These reminders, and the associated emotions, will inspire you to continue your efforts.

Ask daily questions. It's easy to get caught up in the whirlwind of triathlon and forget about why you put so much into the sport. It's easy to begin a workout and go through the motions without connecting your efforts with your goals. To ensure that you keep your "eye on the prize" and maximize your efforts daily, ask yourself two questions. When you get up in the morning, ask, "What can I do today to become the best triathlete I can be?" and before you go to sleep, ask, "Did I do everything possible today to become the best triathlete I can be?" These two questions will remind you daily of what your goal is and will challenge you to be motivated to become your best.

Develop the heart of motivation. Though the techniques we've just described can help increase your motivation, motivation must ultimately come from within. If you have the passion to participate in triathlon, you will be motivated to achieve your goals. Motivation to train and race ultimately surfaces because you love the process of triathlon more than the results. Compete because you just enjoy being out there. If you truly love triathlon, the motivation to pursue your goals will be there when you head out to swim, bike, or run.

TRIATHLETE SPOTLIGHT: MARIA

While growing up, Maria never thought of herself as an athlete. She didn't play organized sports and hated to run. Now squarely in her 30s, she was overweight, out of shape, and beginning to worry about her health. Sadly, her mother recently died of cancer. Maria decided she needed to make some changes in her life, but she didn't know where to begin. While visiting a local sports store in search of a pair of running shoes that she thought might motivate her to begin running, she saw an announcement for the Leukemia and Lymphoma Society Team-in-Training sprint triathlon program, and she had an epiphany. Her mother had taught her to swim as a child, and she always liked to ride her bike in her neighborhood. And Maria wanted some way to pay tribute to her mother and to help others with cancer.

As the TnT training program got under way, Maria regularly told herself how stupid she was to think that she could finish a triathlon. Training was tiring, and she was always sore. She thought of quitting each day, but whenever that thought crossed her mind, she thought of her mother and how wonderful it would feel to cross the finish line in her honor. Maria knew how proud her mother would be for what she was doing. Whenever she was in her kitchen, Maria would look at a photo of her mother, feel her love, and become overwhelmed with the pride and inspiration she felt with her TnT efforts. The coaches, mentors, and "TnTers" were also so positive and supportive, telling her how much she was improving. And she was having a really good time, making new friends and getting more fit.

As the weeks of training passed, the discomfort of training lessened and Maria actually looked forward to her workouts. She was losing weight and feeling better than ever. She went so far as to set a time goal for her

(continued on next page)

(continued from previous page)

first triathlon. As race day approached, she was a bit scared, but she was ready to race for her mother. The race itself was a blast for her. Everyone was cheering for the TnTers, and she felt like everyone in the race was behind her. Her mother was with her every step of the way. Near the end, it really hurt, but knowing the finish line wasn't far off inspired her to keep going. Maria crossed the line to see that she didn't quite reach her time goal, but she didn't care. She had done something that she never thought possible, and she cried for both joy and sadness, thinking how happy her mother would be with her accomplishment. The next day, she signed up to be a mentor for the next TnT triathlon training program.

4 Confidence

Confidence is the most important mental contributor to triathlon success. We define confidence as how strongly you believe you can perform your best and achieve your goals. Confidence affects every aspect of your training, your competitive performances, and your life in general. You may have the ability to achieve your triathlon goals, but if you don't believe you have that ability, then you won't perform to the level at which you're physically capable. For example, you may have the fitness to run a 48-minute 10K at the end of an Olympic-distance race, but you won't run at that pace if you don't have the confidence that you can successfully maintain that pace for the entire distance.

Though the best triathletes in the world may have greater strength, speed, and stamina than others, it is their profound belief in their ability to perform against the strongest field of competitors, under the most difficult conditions, in the biggest race of their lives that enables them to be successful. These triathletes believe they can push their limits and achieve their goals. Less self-assured triathletes may not have the confidence to pick up the pace on the ride or put on a surge during the run, believing that they can't maintain that advantage to the finish.

Maintaining confidence is challenging in triathlon because there are so many different types of fitness, skills, and conditions that you must train for and confront in training and races. In addition to the overall feelings of confidence you have as a triathlete, you also have some level of confidence for each part of the sport. You may have a great deal of confidence in your swimming and running, but have serious doubts about your cycling. You may be positive about flat run courses, but unsure of hills. The complexity of triathlon requires you to not only have a comprehensive training program, but also the means to build your confidence in all of these areas.

VICIOUS CYCLE OR UPWARD SPIRAL

Confidence not only influences performance directly, it also affects every other mental factor. To help illustrate the impact of confidence on you as a triathlete, recall a time when you didn't have confidence in your triathlon ability. You may have been caught in a vicious cycle of low confidence and performance in which negative thinking led to poor performance, which led to more negative thinking and even poorer performance. Conversely, remember a time when you were supremely confident. You were likely caught in an upward spiral in which great confidence led to improved performance, which resulted in even more confidence and even higher performance.

Vicious Cycle

The vicious cycle may start with a period of poor training or a bad race. You get discouraged and begin to question your fitness and your ability to achieve your goals. You think and talk negatively: "I'm in terrible shape. I won't do well in this weekend's race." You lose your motivation to train because you assume you'll have bad workouts.

You get nervous before races because you expect to do poorly. All of that anxiety hurts your confidence because you feel physically uncomfortable and there's no way you can race well when you're so uptight. The negative self-talk and anxiety cause negative emotions. You feel frustrated, angry, and helpless, all of which hurt your confidence more and cause you to perform even worse.

All of this negativity hurts your focus. You focus on all of the negatives rather than on things that will help you to train and race well. The negative thoughts, anxiety, bad emotions, and poor focus cause you to feel even more pain than usual. Every part of training and racing is more difficult because your mind and body are more vulnerable to pain. If you're thinking negatively, caught in a vicious cycle, feeling nervous, depressed, and frustrated, unfocused, and in pain, you're not going to feel motivated to train or perform well.

Upward Spiral

Recall when you have been confident in your abilities. You have complete faith that you can achieve your goals. Your self-talk is positive: "I'm feeling really fit. I'm going to have a great race." The positive talk motivates you to give your best effort, allowing you to feel prepared, relaxed, and energized at races. You have positive emotions, such as excitement, inspiration, and pride. You focus on positive aspects of your performance and you're not distracted. The positive thoughts, feelings of calm, sharp focus, and good emotions allow you to feel less pain in training and races. If you're thinking positively, caught in an upward spiral, feeling relaxed and focused, filled with good emotions, and feeling little pain, training and races are more fun and your performances will be strong. The significance of an upward spiral is that every positive factor supports and bolsters the others, so that you think, feel, and perform well throughout your workouts and races.

> *I never dealt with a negative place. I didn't think about things that could go wrong; if something went wrong I would handle it. I kept my mind always on the positive, only on the positive.*
>
> —Mike Pigg,
> winningest triathlete in history

WHY TRIATHLETES LOSE CONFIDENCE

Anything that counters your belief in your ability or suggests that the belief is unfounded will hurt your confidence. Confidence can be hurt by technical breakdowns, tactical errors, equipment failures, a bad day of training, or a poor race result. These setbacks can communicate that you may not be as capable as you thought you were.

Unrealistic expectations can also hurt confidence. Be sure that your confidence is realistic. In other words, is your confidence in your ability consistent with your actual ability? If not, then you may have unrealistic expectations. If you're a perfectionist—as many triathletes are—you're particularly vulnerable to losing confidence because your expectations may be too high. These unrealistic expectations can set you up for failure. If you're overly critical of your performances due to unreasonable expectations, you may believe that you didn't perform as well as you should have, when you may have performed well compared to reasonable expectations.

Lack of experience or skills can also hurt confidence. If you're a newbie or you're new to a particular distance, you may not have the experience to adequately judge how well you should perform. Often, performances that are interpreted as poor are actually just due to the new challenges you're facing at the new distance. You may simply lack the experience to be performing as well as you would like at this point. An inability to adjust your perceptions so they're consistent with your experience may cause a decline in confidence.

PRIME CONFIDENCE

Prime confidence is a deep, lasting, and resilient belief in your ability to achieve your triathlon goals. With prime confidence, you have a solid faith in yourself as a triathlete. You're able to stay confident even when you're having a poor training day, are tired, sick, injured, or having a bad race. Prime confidence keeps you positive, motivated, intense, focused, and emotionally in control. With prime confidence, you respect the challenges you're faced with, but you're not intimidated. Prime confidence also encourages you to seek out difficult conditions and courses and to view them as opportunities to demonstrate your capabilities, not threats to avoid. Prime confidence enables you to perform at your highest level consistently.

> *I remember in '84 [at Hawaii Ironman®], when Mark [Allen] had a twelve-minute lead on the bike. I remember thinking, "He's doing something that is very uncomfortable" and when I was getting splits and saw that he was consistently ahead by twelve minutes, I was in disbelief. On the run we were matching splits, and in the back of my mind I thought, "Mark can't hold this pace; it's superhuman." I just knew. Now it's nine minutes, then six minutes and I thought—"I've got him. I've got him now."*
>
> —Dave Scott

Prime confidence is a belief, not a certainty, that you can achieve your goals. It's the confidence that, if you're well trained, race ready, execute an intelligent plan, and are mentally prepared, you will achieve your goals. Prime confidence reflects faith and trust in your ability and your preparation, and allows you to stay focused on the positive experience of training and racing.

PROGRESSION OF CONFIDENCE

What makes a Simon Lessing or Siri Lindley great champions? What is noticeable about them and other top triathletes is their unwavering belief in their ability to succeed. Whether you're a pro, a committed age grouper, or a first-time triathlete, in addition to building the fitness to be successful, you want to develop strong and resilient confidence to perform at your highest level and achieve your goals.

A question we're often asked is, "Do I become confident by succeeding or do I succeed from being confident?" Our answer is, both. You don't move from 0-percent confidence to 100-percent confidence in one big step. Rather, it's a building process, much like the process of gaining physical fitness; confidence leads to success, which reinforces the confidence, which in turn leads to more success. For example, you may be only 40-percent confident that you can ride a half-Ironman bike segment in under four hours. By working on your cycling fitness and riding technique, and using the confidence-building techniques described in the following pages, your confidence goes up to 60 percent. With your confidence now at 60 percent, you are able to have better-quality rides, which result in improved conditioning and technique, increased cardio-

When I was in a race and my legs felt dreadful, I had to remind myself that I've had lots of runs like this, lots of training like this. Then I would start to come out of it; a shift would happen. It would be a power shift in confidence.

—Dave Scott

vascular efficiency, and faster riding times. Your hard work and progress raise your confidence to 80 percent. Your improved preparation and greater confidence results in better performances in shorter-distance early-season races. Your improved training and race performances then increase your confidence to near 100 percent, enabling you to enter your target half-Ironman race with the confidence that you can achieve your time goal.

Below we have identified five strategies that will help you build a solid foundation of confidence. These approaches involve creating an environment that will allow you to gain confidence in a steady and progressive way. They also require that you take active steps to develop your confidence in all parts of your training so that this confidence emerges in your races.

Preparation Breeds Confidence

Preparation is the foundation of confidence. If you believe that you have done everything you can to perform your best—put in the hours swimming, riding, running, strengthening, and stretching—you will have confidence in your ability to achieve your goals. This preparation includes the physical, technical, tactical, and mental parts of triathlon. If you've developed these areas as fully as you can, you will have faith at the start line that you are as ready as you can be.

Preparation offers you the opportunity to establish trust in your capabilities. As you overcome the many physical, technical, and mental challenges of training, you begin to believe that you can achieve your goals. An important part of gaining this trust is recognizing your efforts. At the end of every workout, stop and reflect on what you accomplished in terms of the specifics of the workouts; the determination, effort, focus, and intensity required to complete a difficult workout; and how the training session has taken you one step closer to your goals. Foster further confidence by acknowledging the progress you're making. Seeing and feeling yourself gain strength, speed, and stamina will steadily boost your confidence.

Mental Skills Reinforce Confidence

Mental skills that strengthen and maintain motivation, confidence, intensity, focus, and emotions, and lessen pain can be thought of as tools from your triathlon toolbox you can use when faced with challenges in your training and races. These challenges may come from external forces, for example, the weather, terrain, or distance. You can use mental skills to ensure that you view these challenges positively, and stay motivated, focused, relaxed, and emotionally upbeat. Other challenges can be internal, such as fatigue and pain. When your body is struggling, you can use mental skills to help your mind to encourage your body to keep going and to master the pain. Mental skills give you the tools you need to respond positively to these external and internal challenges. Common mental skills you can put in your toolbox (that will be discussed throughout this book) include goal setting to bolster motivation, positive self-talk to maintain confidence, intensity control to stay relaxed, keywords to maintain focus and avoid distractions, emotional control to stay calm when things aren't going well, and pain control to combat discomfort at the end of a race.

Adversity Ingrains Confidence

Having confidence in your ability to complete a triathlon within your desired time goal isn't enough. You need to also develop a belief that you can overcome the many forms of adversity that are a normal part of triathlon racing—cold and rough water and bumping against others in the swim; hills, headwinds, and flat tires on the bike; and heat, sore legs, blisters, and fatigue on the run. Your biggest challenge is to maintain your confidence when faced with adversity. The primary way to gain this confidence in the face of adversity is to expose yourself to adversity in training.

We all love to train when the open water is calm, the rides are without wind, and the runs are flat. If the training conditions are difficult, you may be tempted to shorten or skip the workout entirely. Race conditions are, however, rarely ideal. Training under adverse conditions allows you to prepare yourself for responding positively to race adversity. Tough conditions will then feel familiar and more comfortable, and they won't prevent you from giving your best effort.

Working out in adverse conditions has several benefits. It allows you to feel tough, confident, and inspired during your training. You'll be able to practice how you can respond to similar conditions in races—positive self-talk, staying relaxed and focused. You will gain valuable experience in dealing with the adversity in terms of technique, tactics, nutrition, and other race-related factors, better preparing you for those conditions in races. Finally, when faced with adverse conditions in races, you won't be shocked, dismayed, or defeated by them. Instead, you'll say, "Been there, done that, no big deal," and have the confidence and the tools to overcome the adversity and have a great race.

Overcoming obstacles during racing gives me confidence—some of the best confidence builders are those races that didn't necessarily go as planned but where I pushed through the physical and mental obstacles I faced and crossed the finish line.

—Heather Fuhr

Support Bolsters Confidence

Whether you belong to a triathlon club, a privately coached training group, or you just have a few buddies you work out with, the social aspects of triathlon are also an important source of confidence. This support can foster your confidence in several ways. Training with other triathletes who are positive and motivated is contagious. If you're with upbeat and passionate people, it's hard not to feel the same. You may also receive positive feedback from those with whom you train: "Great work!" "Nice effort today." When other triathletes show confidence in you, you're reminded of the progress you're making and this reinforces your own growing confidence in yourself.

Support for your triathlon involvement may also come from people outside of the triathlon community. Getting support from your family is key, particularly if you have significant family responsibilities (e.g., raising children). Finding time to train without sacrificing other parts of your life is a challenge, especially for longer-distance races. Receiving support and encouragement to pursue your triathlon goals can build confidence and reduce stress. Similar support from your coworkers, where you might need flexible hours in order to train, and from friends, who must be forgiving of you for periodically making your training a priority over social activities, can also bolster your confidence.

This support is particularly important after a difficult workout, a low point in your training, or a bad race. Getting support from other triathletes can act as a lifeline that can save you from those confidence-crushing episodes. A few well-chosen words, a pat on the back, or a hug from your coach, training partners, or a family member can get you out of a funk, put your situation in perspective, safeguard your confidence, and get you back on track. Remember also that support is a two-way street. Just as you get encouragement from others within and outside of the triathlon world, allow yourself to give it to others when the opportunity arises.

> *The best coaches I ever had were my training partners; they knew me well and knew when I was feeling good or not. You need someone who sees you day to day and who knows how your energy rises and falls. Someone who can give you perspective when you can't give it to yourself, and someone who knows what you're going through with your training and racing. You can also learn from your training partners. I used to watch Mark [Allen] a lot when we trained. I learned a lot from that.*
>
> —Paul Huddle,
> former pro triathlete and coach

Success Validates Confidence

All of your efforts to build your confidence are directed toward achieving triathlon success. You may think about success as great races and reaching competitive goals, but success starts in training. Every day that you swim, ride, or run, you're achieving little victories that incrementally bolster your confidence. With each of these small "wins," your confidence steadily grows until you have the confidence to achieve a big "win," such as realizing a previously determined race goal. Because big wins don't come often, the small wins are important for strengthening and maintaining your confidence. To gain the benefits of the little successes, recognize them when they occur. After every workout, be sure to acknowledge the small victories. Reflect on how diligently you worked and how you achieved your day's training goals.

These small victories generate positive emotions, such as inspiration, pride, excitement, fulfillment, and happiness, rooting your confidence more deeply in your psyche. Combining your belief in your ability

When my results started to get better, I began to actually believe in myself and my abilities. Only then did I have the confidence to toe the line and believe that I could compete with the best.

—Heather Fuhr

with powerful, positive emotions makes your confidence stronger and more resilient. This resilience comes from you making these small deposits in your "confidence bank." With a big confidence balance, you'll be able to make withdrawals on challenging training or race days. Training success rewards your efforts—"All that hard work really paid off"—encouraging you to continue to strive toward your triathlon goals. Ultimately, the small victories set the stage for a big success (in the form of achieving a race goal) and fully validate the confidence that you have so patiently developed.

CONFIDENCE IS A SKILL

Confidence is a skill, much like technical skills, that you can develop through practice and experience. One problem you may have is that you've developed poor confidence skills. By being negative and not believing in yourself, you may become very skilled at being negative, which hurts your ability to perform. For example, if you've developed a bad technical habit, such as a poor recovery in your swim stroke, you will be skilled at that poor stroke motion. That bad habit will then come out in a race and cause you to swim more slowly than you are capable. The same holds true for confidence. You can become skilled at being negative, and that bad habit can come out in races and hurt your confidence and your race performances.

To change bad confidence habits, you must retrain the way you think. You have to practice good confidence skills regularly until the old negative habits have been broken and you've learned and ingrained the new positive skills of confidence. The techniques described below will help you in this process by giving you specific strategies you can use to unlearn bad habits and learn effective confidence skills.

Positive Self-talk

In addition to the five confidence-building strategies we just described, there is one more technique that is a powerful tool to maintain and strengthen your confidence in training and races. This secret weapon is *positive self-talk*. What you say to yourself when you're in the pool, on your bike, or in your running shoes affects what you think, how you feel, and how you perform. It may also determine the quality of your workouts and your race results. Whichever form of self-talk you most use—whether positive or negative—will affect your attitude toward your training and races.

Negative self-talk involves thinking or saying anything that reflects a lack of confidence and a defeatist attitude, for example, "I'm going to do lousy today," "I stink," or "I can't deal with these conditions." You may hear it during group training regularly. It can suck the life and love out of training and races. You may also participate in the negative self-talk. If you say these things to yourself, you're convincing yourself that you have little chance. With a negative attitude your mind may counter your efforts, your motivation will wane, you'll lose focus, and you'll experience much more pain. By using positive self-talk, for example, "I can deal with these conditions" and "I am strong and prepared," your attitude will translate into prime confidence, intensity, focus, and helpful emotions, and will result in a great performance.

Positive self-talk increases your motivation to work hard because you believe that your efforts will be rewarded. You're relaxed and focused because you believe you can handle anything that is thrown at you by the course and the weather. Your emotions reflect and increase your positive self-talk with feelings of excitement and joy. Most importantly, positive self-talk helps keep your mind strong and your body moving toward the finish line, especially when your body is tired and in pain. As your body wears down late in workouts and races, it will communicate to your mind that it has had enough—"I get the point! You can stop now." Positive self-talk can help your mind persuade your body to keep going.

Positive self-talk is most valuable when you think your tank is empty. Unless you're having a Julie Moss moment (recalling her unforgettable 1982 Hawaii Ironman® experience when her body simply gave out and only a supreme and inspiring effort enabled her to crawl the last 100 yards and cross the finish line), there is always something left. Positive self-talk is the only thing that can take you from where you think there is nothing left to where there is nothing left. Positive self-talk is your greatest tool against fatigue and pain. It will allow you to tap into that final reserve at the end of a race. If you can say, "Keep at it. This is what I've worked for. I will not give up," then your body will listen and respond.

You need to talk to yourself a lot! When you start to find yourself daydreaming or dwelling on the pain, you have to make a good effort to think positive thoughts.

—Lisa Bentley,
multiple Ironman winner

Training positive self-talk. Positive self-talk is a simple strategy. You replace your negative self-talk with a positive statement. The difficulty lies in overcoming ingrained negative self-talk habits. You begin retraining your self-talk by looking at the situations in which you tend to become negative, for example, when you have to do a cold, open-water swim, ride into a headwind, or run a challenging track workout (see the Know Your Self-Talk form on page 49).

Figure out why you become negative in these situations. Common reasons include fatigue, boredom, pain, frustration, and despair. All triathletes have "hot-button" issues that trigger negativity. Finding out what yours are is essential to changing your self-talk. Then, monitor what you say to yourself. We've found that triathletes tend to rely on favorite negative self-talk when their buttons get pushed, for example, "Gosh, I suck," "You're such a loser," and "What's the point of even trying?" Realizing what you say and how bad it is for you is an important step in changing your self-talk. For most of the triathletes we've worked with, there is a consistent pattern of the situations in which negative self-talk arises, the causes of the negativity, and the specific self-talk they express.

Before you go out and face those hot-button situations again, choose some positive self-talk with which you can replace your usual negative self-talk. The positive self-talk should be encouraging, but it must also be realistic. If you say things like, "I love being out here" when you really don't or "I'm feeling so strong" even when you're not, it's difficult to believe what you're saying. Acknowledging the hot button, but putting a positive and realistic spin on it, will make it more likely you'll believe what you're saying, for example, "If I keep working hard, good things will happen" and "This really hurts, but it's money in the bank for my race." By putting this new tool in your toolbox before your buttons get pushed, you'll have more ready access to responding positively.

Ingraining positive self-talk depends on your ongoing commitment to this process. Because you may be skilled at negative self-talk, you'll have to constantly remind yourself to be positive. Realizing when the hot-button situations are approaching will prepare you to focus on what you say when it happens. At first you may "fall off the wagon" and slip back to your old, negative ways. Accept it as part of the process and return to being positive. With time and persistence, you'll see a gradual shift away from negativity and toward positive self-talk. One workout you'll realize that you just went through one of those hot-button situations and you stayed positive.

Balance the scales. When we work with triathletes, we have them keep track of the number of positive and negative things they say during training and races. In most cases, the negatives far outnumber the positives. In an ideal world, we would eliminate all negatives and only express positives. But if you care about triathlon at all, you may at times think negatively.

> *I'd see people up the road, but I'd never seem to catch them. Today was one of those days you say to yourself, "I can't do this! It's too hard!" You keep thinking of when you're going to stop. It's a matter of talking to yourself and saying "Hey, I've got to keep going on. You can't DNF. You've got to give it everything you've got." I'd have been happy if I had finished 100th and known I'd given it my all.*
>
> —Lori Bowden,
> 2003 Ironman world champion

KNOW YOUR SELF-TALK

Directions: In the space below, list the situations in which you tend to use negative self-talk, the causes of the negativity, the common negative thoughts that you have, and positive replacements.

	Hot-Button Situation	Hot-Button Cause	Negative Self-Talk	Positive Replacement
1.				
2.				
3.				
4.				

In dealing with this reality, learn to balance the scales. The immediate goal is to increase the positives. If you're negative when you perform poorly, be positive when you do well. If you beat yourself up over a bad swim, pat yourself on the back for a good ride. Tell yourself "nice effort" when you gave a nice effort. Give yourself a "job well done" when you've done the job well.

Once you've balanced the scales by increasing your positives, your next goal is to tip the scales in the positive direction by reducing the negatives. Ask why you're so hard on yourself when you perform poorly. Acknowledge that the process of success for triathletes of all levels involves difficulties and lessons learned. The down periods are an integral part of that learning process.

This step of tipping the scales toward positives is critical. Recent research found that negative experiences such as negative self-talk, negative body language, and negative emotions carry more weight than positive experiences. In fact, it takes twelve positive experiences to equal one negative experience. What this means is that for every negative expression you make about yourself, whether saying something negative or screaming in frustration, you must express yourself positively twelve times to counteract that one negative expression.

Your goal is to tip the scale heavily in the positive direction. Sure, you're going to say some negative things periodically. That's just part of being human and being a triathlete. You get tired, sick, and injured. You get frustrated, angry, and depressed. The conditions get the better of you. So you get down on yourself once in a while. Your goal is to respond positively most of the time to the situations that used to push your buttons.

Positive keywords. Another useful way to develop your confidence is to use keywords that remind you to be positive and confident. Make a list of words that make you feel optimistic and positive. Then write them on your equipment, for example, on your handlebars, where they're visible during training and races. Put keywords in noticeable places where you live, such as in your bedroom, on your refrigerator door, or in your locker. When you look at a keyword, say it to yourself. Every time you see it, it will sink in further until you truly believe it.

Using negative thinking positively. As we just mentioned, we emphasize being positive at all times but realize that this is challenging. This awareness was brought home at a USA Triathlon junior-elite training camp at which Jim worked. During the camp, he was constantly emphasizing to the athletes to be positive and not negative. One night at dinner, several of the triathletes came up to him and said that sometimes things do just stink and you can't be positive. He realized that negative thinking is natural when you don't perform well. It means you care about performing poorly and want to do better. Negative thinking can be motivating by impelling you to want to improve. Jim got to thinking about how triathletes could use negative thinking in a positive way. He came up with an important distinction that will determine whether negative thinking helps or hurts your triathlon efforts.

There are two types of negative thinking: give-up negative thinking and fire-up negative thinking. Give-up negative thinking involves feelings of despair, helplessness, and loss, for example, "It's over. I can't finish." You dwell on past mistakes and failures. It hurts your motivation and confidence and takes your focus away from continuing to give your best effort. Your intensity also drops because you're surrendering and accepting defeat. There is never a place in triathlon for give-up negative thinking.

In contrast, fire-up negative thinking involves feelings of anger and energy, of being psyched up, for example, "I'm doing so badly. I hate performing this way!" You look to doing better in the future because you dislike performing poorly. Fire-up negative thinking increases your motivation to fight and turn things around. Your intensity goes up and you're bursting with energy. Fire-up negative thinking can be a positive way to turn your performance around. But remember, negative thinking and negative emotions require a lot of energy that could be put to better use in your training and races, so don't use it for too long.

Recognize Your Strengths and Weaknesses

Many triathletes have a difficult time seeing their strengths. Because there is such a strong sense of social comparison in triathlon—there is always someone who is stronger, faster, and has better endurance—you may see yourself as paling in comparison. But regardless of how you stack up against others, you have strengths that you can rely on to achieve your goals. But your strengths won't help you unless you acknowledge them. Take a close look at what you bring to triathlon and identify your strengths in terms of the range of abilities you have to succeed. Recognizing your strengths will bolster your confidence. You'll admit that you have qualities that you can use to perform well. Commit to developing your strengths even further so they have an even greater effect on your performances. As your awareness of your strengths solidifies, you gain more confidence that they will help you achieve your goals.

Knowing your strengths is only half the battle. Acknowledge your weaknesses as well. Though admitting your weaknesses may feel like a blow to your ego, it is an essential part of building confidence and achieving your triathlon goals. By knowing your weaknesses you can take steps to improve them and turn them into strengths. If you're not a very good climber on your bike, ride hills. If you make climbing a priority in your training, you will become more capable and confident with this challenge. While working on those weaknesses, your confidence will rise along with your fitness. Whether your efforts result in turning your weaknesses into strengths or simply minimizing how much your weaknesses hurt your performance depends on your genetics and how much time and effort you put into overcoming your weaknesses. In either case, you'll have much more confidence in your weaknesses than ever before.

Positive Body Language

One thing we've noticed about working with professional and top age-group triathletes is that they carry themselves a certain way. They move and walk with confidence. Another way to develop your confidence is to learn to "walk the walk." How you carry yourself, move, and walk affects what you think and how you feel. If your body is down, your thoughts and feelings will be negative. If your body is up, your thoughts and feelings will be positive. It's hard to feel down when your body is up. Positive body language involves keeping your head high, chin up, eyes forward, shoulders back, arms swinging, and a bounce in your step. You look and move like a winner.

Be Optimistic

Optimistic people are positive, upbeat, "glass half full" kind of people. Not surprisingly, optimism is significantly related to athletic success; the more optimistic people are, the better they perform. There are some good reasons for this relationship. Optimists tend to be confident and positive when they're faced with challenges. They see difficulties, for example, rough water, a hilly bike course, or a hot training run, as opportunities to push themselves, gain experience, and improve as triathletes. Even when things are going badly, optimists find constructive challenges in the adversity that they can use to stay positive and motivated. They tend to persevere when faced with demanding situations. "Give up" is simply not a part of their vocabulary. Optimists bounce back following poor performances. Because they believe things will turn out well, optimists maintain their efforts and stay positive, relaxed, and focused. This state of mind with all of its side benefits sustains them at the worst of times. This hopefulness encourages them to challenge themselves and get out of their comfort zone. Though they may not always succeed, optimists are willing, for example, to try swimming in a faster lane at masters, hang with the lead group on a ride, or stay with faster runners at the track.

You may be thinking, "Sure, it would be great to be an optimist, but I wasn't born one and everyone knows that you either have it or you don't." Our response to you is: "Wrong!" Though some people do seem to be born optimists, optimism can be learned. It just takes practice. You can become more optimistic by using the many confidence-building strategies we discuss in this chapter and slowly tipping the scales of your attitude in a positive direction.

It isn't quite that easy though. Pessimism has protective value in that when things do go poorly it simply confirms what you expected would happen. If you don't get your hopes up or expect too much, you can't be that disappointed. But the downside to pessimism is that you

For years I have been asked how much a great triathlon performance can be attributed to attitude. My answer is always the same—on race day, it's all about attitude. Its value in improving performance should not be underestimated.

—Mark Allen,
six-time Ironman world champion

may never free yourself to take a risk or face a new challenge. It also means that you can never perform to the very best of your ability or experience the joy of having given it your all. Being a pessimist is safe and comfortable, but ultimately frustrating and unsatisfying.

For you to become more optimistic, you have to take a leap of faith. This leap means saying, "To heck with it. I'm just going to give it everything I've got and see what happens." Your past experiences and basic beliefs may not support your leap, but you're going to jump anyway. The chances are, if you're at all prepared to achieve your goals, you will succeed. This success will affirm your leap of faith and make your next leap easier and less scary. As you take more leaps of faith you'll gain more confidence that positive results will occur in the future. You'll become more optimistic and hopeful. Before you know it, you'll look at every challenging situation and tough condition and believe—optimistically—that you will overcome them and achieve your goals.

Confidence Challenge

The real test of confidence is how you respond when things are not going your way. We call this the Confidence Challenge. It's easy to stay confident when you're healthy and rested and the conditions are ideal. But as we said earlier, an inevitable part of triathlon is that you'll have some down periods or be faced with adversity. Consistently successful triathletes are able to maintain their confidence when things are difficult. By staying confident, they persevere rather than give up, and they know that, in time, their performance will come around.

Triathletes with prime confidence seek out ways to minimize the down periods and return to their optimal level. All triathletes will go through periods when they don't perform well. The skill is to get out of the down periods quickly. The Confidence Challenge is a mental skill that you can develop to help you out of those ruts. Learning to respond positively to the Confidence Challenge comes from exposing yourself to demanding situations and difficult conditions in training and races and practicing positive responses.

Confidence allows you to take risks. Risks allow you to be confident and will give you breakthrough performances. Without risks and challenges you may not believe you can press forward. Confidence gives you the belief you can.

—Victor Plata,
2004 U.S. Olympic Triathlon Team

There are several key aspects of mastering the Confidence Challenge. First, develop the attitude that demanding situations are challenges to be sought out rather than threats to be avoided. When you're faced with a Confidence Challenge, see it as an opportunity to become a better triathlete. Believe that experiencing challenges is a necessary part of becoming the best triathlete you can be. At first, these challenges may be uncomfortable due to their difficulty and unfamiliarity. But as you expose yourself to more challenges, they will become less threatening and more comfortable.

With this perspective, seek out every possible challenge in training and races. Be sure you're well prepared to meet the challenges. Mastering the Confidence Challenge requires the physical fitness and mental skills to do so. Stay positive and motivated in the face of difficulties. Focus on what you need to do to overcome the challenge rather than focusing on how thorny it may be. Accept that you may struggle at first when faced with a new challenge. View these experiences as lessons you can draw from when faced with those challenges again. Finally, and most importantly, never, ever give up!

TRIATHLETE SPOTLIGHT: CARY

Cary, a 26-year-old middle-of-the-packer in Olympic-distance races, was his own worst enemy, not only in triathlon, but in most parts of his life. He often expected the worst and, not surprisingly, the worst is what usually happened. In training, when things got hard, he would get down on himself and constantly ask himself what the heck he was doing out there. In races, as soon as he started feeling some pain, his mind would turn against him and he would always slow up. He didn't like being a "downer," but he figured that was the way it was and there wasn't anything he could do about it.

One day, Cary attended a talk on sport psychology sponsored by his local tri-club. The speaker explained how important confidence was and, if you were negative, how it was possible to turn it around and become more positive. Tired of his negativity, he decided to give the speaker's ideas a try, though, characteristically, he didn't expect them to work.

Over the next week of training, he paid attention to his self-talk and what he said to others during training. After each workout, he wrote down the negative and positive things he remembered saying. Even he was shocked at how negative he was. In a week's worth of training, he recalled thinking or saying ninety-seven negative things and only four positive ones.

The first thing he did was to make a list of the situations in which he typically got negative. He noticed that most of his negativity occurred later in workouts and races when he started to get tired and started to hurt. He realized that he usually eased up or even gave up when that happened. He then wrote down some positive things he could say to himself when he began to feel that way.

Over the next few weeks, Cary committed himself to being more positive, but it was a real struggle. Negative stuff would just pop into his head and, when he tried to be positive, his negative thoughts would take over again. It was as if there were two sides to him—Dr. Jekyll and Mr. Hyde—

(continued on next page)

(continued from previous page)

and they were battling it out for control. Keeping daily records of his self-talk, after the first week, his positive-to-negative ratio was still really low, 21 to 76, but that was an improvement. As his workouts continued, he noticed that being positive was becoming easier, his training efforts were better, and he was enjoying training more. After a month, he finally turned the corner, calculating that his positive-to-negative ratio was 44 to 21, still not stellar, but heading in the right direction, and a month later, his ratio was up to 76 to 10. But the real test would be in his upcoming Olympic-distance race.

For the first time in a while, Cary was actually excited about the race. Through the early part of the race, he felt good and had little negativity. With about three miles to go in the run, he started to hurt. As usual, negatives began to pop up, but he immediately countered them with positive self-talk. Though certainly not a ton of fun, he kept positive to the end and, for the first time ever, sprinted the last quarter mile to the finish line. He had a great race and, feeling flushed with pride, an even better attitude. He turned to a teammate and said, "This mental stuff actually works."

5 Intensity

Whether you're aware of it or not, your intensity has an enormous influence on your training and race efforts. Intensity is the feeling of adrenaline and energy that's radiating from you before a sprint-distance race. It is the raw nerves of anxiety and apprehension that you feel from the nearly 2,000 competitors before the start of an Ironman. Intensity is the feeling of calm and relaxation that you see among the pro triathletes before the swim. It is the excitement and exhilaration you feel as you transition from the bike to the run. And it is the relief you experience crossing the finish line after a hard race.

Intensity in triathlon has a complex and conflicting nature. It can help or hurt your ability to perform your best. It can feel powerful and positive or uncomfortable and negative. Even more confusing, intensity that is unpleasant is sometimes necessary for achieving your goals and intensity that feels good doesn't always translate into a great performance.

Intensity is one of the most important contributors to triathlon performance immediately before and once the race begins. It's so important because being completely mentally prepared won't help you if your body is not physiologically capable of doing what it needs to do for you to perform your best. Intensity sets the tone for the motivation, confidence, focus, and emotions you will carry into your race. It may also affect how readily you can access the mental skills that you've developed in training and need to use in your races. And it will affect the pain you experience during your triathlon efforts.

Intensity is made up of two components. The first is what you feel physically, that is, what you actually feel in your body before and during races. Intensity is the amount of physiological activity you experience in your body, including heart rate, blood flow, respiration, and adrenaline. Are you calm or nervous, relaxed or tense? Intensity lies on a continuum ranging from sleep (very relaxed) to terror (highly anxious). Somewhere in between these two extremes is the level of intensity at which you perform your best. One of the confounding aspects of intensity is that there isn't one ideal level of intensity for all triathletes or all race distances. Some triathletes perform best very relaxed, others moderately intense, and still others very intense. Shorter-distance races, as a rule, require higher intensity because speed is needed. Because intensity is energy that needs to be conserved, much like gasoline in your automobile's fuel tank, longer races call for lower intensity. If you burn too much fuel too early, you'll run out of gas before the finish. You have to figure the level of intensity at which you perform best in the different distance events.

The second component involves your perception of intensity. Do you perceive intensity positively or negatively? Does it feel comfortable or distressing? Two triathletes can feel the exact same thing physiologically, but interpret those physical feelings in very different ways. One may view the intensity as excitement that will aid performance while another may see the intensity as anxiety that may hurt performance.

The physical experience and the perception of intensity are affected by several mental factors. If you're not confident, feeling frustrated and angry, focusing on winning rather than on performing, and in pain, you may see your intensity as negative. In contrast, if you're confident and positive, happy and excited, focused on doing your best, and feeling little discomfort, you'll view your intensity positively. Conversely, your intensity will influence these factors as well, for example, if you're optimally intense, you'll likely have more confidence, experience positive emotions, focus well, and feel less pain.

I am very fired up mentally when the gun goes off. I may be calm and cool outside, but inside it's like a cannon goes off when the gun sounds. I am ready to bring everything I have mentally and physically to the table.

—Pete Kain

OVERINTENSITY AND UNDERINTENSITY

Intensity produces a wide array of physical and mental symptoms that can help you recognize when your intensity is too high or too low. These signs are usually obvious, yet you may not notice them because the signs are ever present or you may not realize that they indicate a problem. By being aware of these signs, you'll know when you're not performing at your optimal intensity and can take steps to reach your ideal level.

Overintensity. Muscle tension and breathing difficulties are the most common signs of overintensity. Many triathletes say that when they're too intense, they feel tension in their neck, shoulders, and legs. If your neck and shoulders are tense during the swim, your swim stroke will shorten and you won't swim with comfort or fluidity. If your torso is tense on the bike, you'll have a less efficient pedal stroke and you will feel uncomfortable in your riding position. When your legs are tense during the run, you lose the ability to run smoothly. Muscle tension causes your shoulders and your center of gravity to rise, reducing your power on the bike and your stride length on the run. Overintensity can also disrupt coordination, lowering your efficiency in all three legs of a triathlon.

Many triathletes also report that their breathing becomes short and choppy when nervous. This restriction in breathing is a natural reaction to stress, but it limits the intake of oxygen that is necessary for endurance. Constrained breathing means that your body won't work efficiently, you won't be able to maintain your pace, you're more likely to cramp, and you will tire more quickly. In addition, the smoothness of your movements will tend to mirror your breathing in all three triathlon events. If your breathing is long and smooth, your stroke, cadence, and stride will be as well. If your breathing is abrupt and choppy, your movements will be jerky and uncomfortable. When you're overly intense, you may also exhibit poor posture and a stiff gait.

Overintensity can hurt you mentally as well. Anxiety lowers confidence and causes doubts about your ability—"If I'm nervous, I must not be prepared for the race." The physical and mental discomfort of overintensity may produce negative emotions, such as frustration and anger. The anxiety, doubts, and negative emotions hurt focus by drawing your attention away from performing your best. Overintensity can also interfere with clear thinking, causing technical or tactical errors throughout the race.

Underintensity. Though not as common, you may also experience underintensity before and during races. The most frequent symptoms of underintensity are low energy and lethargy. You lack the energy and "giddyap" you need to give your best effort. Though not as uncomfortable as overintensity, underintensity hurts your performance equally because you lack the physical requisites, including sufficient heart rate, respiration, blood flow, and adrenaline, to achieve your goals. Without sufficient intensity, strength and endurance will be less than optimal.

Mentally, underintensity undermines your confidence, motivation, and focus. You don't have faith in your ability to succeed and you just don't feel like being out there. Your lack of interest created by low intensity causes you to be easily distracted and to have difficulty staying focused on your race.

PRIME INTENSITY

Prime intensity is the ideal amount of physiological activity necessary for you to perform your best. It's also the level of intensity that you perceive as most positive and beneficial to your training and race performances. As we mentioned earlier, there isn't one level of intensity that's ideal for everyone. Your goal is to discover the level of intensity that enables you to perform your best. You have several objectives in developing prime intensity. First, define your prime intensity. Then, recognize the signs of overintensity and underintensity. Next, identify race situations in which your intensity may go up or down. Finally, psych up or psych down to reach and maintain prime intensity throughout a race.

Your intensity is much like a thermostat whose purpose is to maintain the most comfortable temperature in your house. You always notice when your house is too warm or too cold because you're sensitive to changes in temperature. When the temperature becomes uncomfortable, you adjust the thermostat to a more comfortable level. You can think of intensity as your internal temperature that needs to be adjusted periodically. You need to be sensitive to when your intensity is no longer comfortable, in other words, when it's not allowing you to perform well. You can then use the intensity-control techniques described in this chapter to raise or lower your intensity to its prime level.

The ultimate goal of prime intensity is to find the precise line between overintensity or underintensity. Prime intensity is the physiological level at which your body performs well and at which you are most comfortable. If your intensity is too low or too high, your body won't perform at the level to which it is capable. The closer you can get to that line of prime intensity, the better your body will perform. Successful triathletes have the ability to do two things related to intensity. They have a better understanding of where that line of prime intensity is so they can "tightrope walk" on it, thereby maximizing what their bodies can give them in a race. They're also able to stay on that line longer than other triathletes, which enables them to perform at a consistently higher level for longer periods of time.

Determining Prime Intensity

Using the Intensity Identification form (see page 63), you can identify your prime intensity. Think back to several races in which you performed well. Recall your level of intensity. Were you relaxed, energized, or really fired up? Then remember the thoughts, emotions, and physical feelings you experienced during these races. Were you positive or negative, happy or angry, relaxed or tense? Next, think back to several races in which you were disappointed in your performances. Recall your level of intensity. Remember the thoughts, emotions, and physical feelings you had in these competitions. Like most triathletes, a distinct pattern will likely emerge. When you perform well, you have a particular level of intensity. This is your prime intensity. There are also common thoughts, emotions, and physical feelings associated with performing well. In contrast, when you do worse than expected, there is a very different level of intensity, either higher or lower than your prime intensity, and a different set of thoughts, emotions, and physical feelings.

Another useful way to help you understand your prime intensity is to experiment with different levels of intensity in training and see how the differing intensity affects your performance. Here is a good exercise you can use in your swimming, biking, and running workouts to help you identify your prime intensity:

Let's say you're doing three sets of three 100s in the pool to improve your swim speed. The first set will emphasize low intensity. Before you begin, take several slow, deep breaths, relax your muscles, and focus on calming thoughts (e.g., "Easy does it," "Cool and calm"). Throughout the set, stay focused on keeping your body relaxed and calm.

The second set will focus on moderate intensity. Before the set, take a few deep, but more forceful, breaths, move around in the water, and focus on more energetic thoughts (e.g., "Let's go," "Pick it up"). During the set, use a more vigorous mind-set and focus on putting more effort and energy into your strokes.

The final set will highlight high intensity. Before you start, take several deep, forced breaths with special emphasis on a hard and aggressive exhale, move around very actively in the water, and repeat intense self-talk (e.g., "Fire it up," "Get after it"), saying these out loud with energy and force. During the set, maintain an aggressive mind-set and focus on putting everything you have into your swim.

We encourage you to use this exercise for several days so you can see clearly how your intensity influences your performance. You can use similar exercises for your bike and running workouts. As with the Intensity Identification form, you'll probably see a pattern emerge in which you perform better at one of the three levels of intensity. With this knowledge, you'll have a better sense of your prime intensity and can then use that information before and during races to recognize when you're not at prime intensity and when you need to adjust your intensity to a prime level.

PSYCH-DOWN TECHNIQUES

Before and during races, it's natural for your intensity to increase and for you to feel nervous. To perform your best, take active steps to get your intensity back to its prime level. There are several simple techniques you can use to lower your intensity.

Deep breathing. When you experience overintensity, your breathing is one of the first things that's disrupted. It becomes short and choppy and you don't get the oxygen your body needs. Regain control of your breathing by focusing on taking slow, deep breaths.

Deep breathing has several important benefits. It ensures that you get enough oxygen so your body can function. You will relax, feel better, and it will give you a greater sense of control. Your increased comfort allows you to more readily let go of negative thoughts and reestablish your confidence. It will also help you shed negative emotions, such as frustration and despair. Focusing on your breathing helps take your mind off of things that may be interfering with your performance and back onto areas that will enable you to perform.

In short-course races, where the pre-race atmosphere and the race pace tend to be more frenetic than longer-distance events, deep breathing can be especially valuable before the race when you want to stay calm and in

INTENSITY IDENTIFICATION

Directions: In the space below, indicate factors that are related to your best (prime intensity) and worst (overintensity and underintensity) races.

	Best Races	Worst Races
Importance of Race		
Difficulty of Competition		
Race		
Conditions		
Thoughts		
Emotions		
Physical Feelings		

control. It can also help you reduce your intensity as you enter T1 and T2. Heading into a transition, your heart rate is often high and your adrenaline is flowing. As you approach T1 or T2, take several deep breaths to settle your intensity and help you focus on your transition. Deep breaths as you near the transition area will ensure that your body is more relaxed and comfortable, your transition will be smoother and faster, and you'll be better able to establish a solid rhythm in the early part of the bike or run (learn more about intensity in transitions in Chapter 11).

Muscle relaxation. Muscle tension is the most common sign of over-intensity. Before a race, muscle tension is usually caused by pre-race jitters and manifests itself most often in the neck and shoulders. Pre-race muscle tension not only causes discomfort at a point when you're trying to feel calm and confident, but once the race starts, it can inhibit your swim stroke and slow your swim leg. During the bike, muscle tension can arise from a poor position on the bike or spending too much time in your aero bars. On the run, muscle tension is an unwelcome companion caused by increasing fatigue and pain. Your ability to prevent and relieve muscle tension before and during races helps your body stay relaxed and performing well.

There are two effective muscle relaxation techniques you can use before events: passive relaxation and active relaxation. Similar to deep breathing, muscle relaxation is beneficial because it allows you to regain control of your body and to feel more physically comfortable. It also offers the same mental and emotional advantages as deep breathing.

With passive relaxation, imagine that tension is a liquid that fills your muscles, creating physical and mental discomfort. By imagining the "liquid" muscle tension draining from your body, you'll feel more relaxed. Before a race, close your eyes and follow the passive relaxation procedure described on page 66. As you go through the passive relaxation procedure, take your time, focus on your breathing and your muscles, feel the tension leave your body, and, at the end, focus on your overall state of physical relaxation and mental calmness. You can also use passive relaxation during a race, particularly during the bike or run where you often feel tension in your neck and shoulders. Focusing on allowing the tension to drain out of tight muscles can allow you to maintain a relaxed position and stay comfortable to the finish.

Active relaxation is used when your body is very tense and passive relaxation isn't enough. When your intensity is too high and your muscles are tight due to fatigue or pain, it's difficult to just relax them. So instead of trying to relax your muscles, do just the opposite. Tighten them more, then release them. Our muscles work on what is called an opponent-principle process. For example, before a race, your muscle tension might be at an 8, where 1 is totally relaxed and 10 is very tense, but you perform best at a 4. By further tightening your muscles up to a 10, the natural reaction is for your muscles to rebound back past 8 toward a more relaxed 4. So, making your muscles tenser essentially causes them to become more relaxed.

Active relaxation involves tightening and relaxing four major muscle groups: face and neck, arms and shoulders, chest and back, and buttocks and legs. It can also be individualized to focus on specific trouble spots. To prepare for active relaxation, follow the same preparations as we described for passive relaxation. Before a race, use the active relaxation procedure described on page 67. As you do active relaxation, focus on the differences between tension and relaxation, be aware of how you're able to induce a greater feeling of relaxation, and, at the end, focus on your overall state of physical relaxation and mental calmness. You can use active relaxation as a preventive measure to help you stay relaxed before the start of and early in a race. It is also a powerful tool to combat the muscle tension that builds up late in races as fatigue and pain begin to engulf your body. Tightening different muscle groups during the bike and run can help you recognize built-up tension, counter the effects of your body breaking down, and enable you to maintain your form and pace.

> ▼
>
> *I must say that I have never been this relaxed before Hawaii. It is nice to not waste all the extra energy being nervous.*
> —Peter Reid

Another way to counteract muscle tension is by shaking out your limbs periodically before and during a race. Tension, particularly when caused by overintensity or being in the same position for a long time (e.g., aero position, long bike climb, or maintaining the same cadence or stride length for long periods), can cause your body to tense and your center of gravity to rise. When this happens, you lose power on the bike and stride length on the run. Making it a practice of periodically raising and lowering your shoulders, swinging your arms, shaking out your hands, and allowing your body to settle back down will increase your efficiency, comfort, and performance during a race.

Process focus. One of the primary causes of pre-race overintensity is focusing on the outcome. If you're worried about whether you'll have

PASSIVE RELAXATION

Imagine there are drain plugs on the bottom of your feet. When you open them, all the tension will drain out of your body and you will become very, very relaxed. Take a slow, deep breath.

Now, undo those plugs. Feel the tension begin to drain out of your body. Down from the top of your head, past your forehead, your face and neck; you're becoming more and more relaxed. The tension drains out of your jaw and down past your neck. Now your face and neck are warm, relaxed, and comfortable. Take a slow, deep breath.

The tension continues to drain out of your upper body, past your hands and forearms, and out of your upper arms and shoulders. Now your hands, arms, and shoulders are warm and relaxed and comfortable. Take a slow, deep breath.

The tension continues to drain out of your upper body, past your chest and upper back, down past your stomach and lower back, and your upper body is becoming more and more relaxed. There is no more tension left in your upper body. Now your entire upper body is warm and relaxed and comfortable. Take a slow, deep breath.

The tension continues to drain out of your lower body, past your buttocks and down past your thighs and your knees. Your lower body is becoming more and more relaxed. The tension drains out of your calves. There is almost no more tension left in your body and the last bit of tension drains past your ankles, the balls of your feet, and your toes. Now do a brief survey of your body from head to toe to ensure that there is no more tension left in your body. Your entire body is warm and relaxed and comfortable. Now replace the plugs so that no tension can get back in. Take a slow, deep breath. Feel the calm and relaxation envelop you. Enjoy that feeling and remember what it feels like to be completely relaxed.

a good race, for example, beat your training buddies, achieve a goal time, win your age group, or qualify for Kona, you're bound to get nervous. The prospect of failing to perform up to your expectations is threatening and will likely create nervousness. To reduce the anxiety caused by an outcome focus, redirect your focus to the process. A process focus takes your mind off things that cause your overintensity and shifts your focus onto things that will calm you, build your confi-

ACTIVE RELAXATION

When I say tight, I want you to tighten that body part for five seconds; when I say loose, I want you to relax it.

First, your buttocks and legs. Tight . . . loose. Feel the relaxation. Take a slow, deep breath. Once again with the buttocks and legs. Tight . . . loose. The muscles in your buttocks and legs are warm and relaxed. Feel the difference between the states of tension and relaxation in your buttocks and legs. Take a slow, deep breath.

Now your chest and back. Tight . . . loose. Feel the relaxation. Take a slow, deep breath. Once again with the chest and back. Tight . . . loose. The muscles in your chest and back are warm and relaxed. Feel the difference between the states of tension and relaxation in your chest and back. Take a slow, deep breath.

Now your arms and shoulders. Tight . . . loose. Feel the relaxation. Take a slow, deep breath. Once again with the arms and shoulders. Tight . . . loose. The muscles in your arms and shoulders are warm and relaxed. Feel the difference between the states of tension and relaxation in your arms and shoulders. Take a slow, deep breath.

Now your face and neck. Tight . . . loose. Feel the relaxation. Take a slow, deep breath. Once again with the face and neck. Tight . . . loose. The muscles in your face and neck are warm and relaxed. Feel the difference between the states of tension and relaxation in your face and neck. Take a slow, deep breath.

Now every muscle in your body. Be sure that every muscle is as tight as you can get it. Tight . . . loose. Feel the relaxation. Take a slow, deep breath. Once again with your entire body. Tight . . . loose. Every muscle in your body is warm and relaxed. Feel the difference between the states of tension and relaxation in your entire body. Take a slow, deep breath.

Now do a mental checklist to make sure that every muscle is relaxed. Your feet are relaxed, calves, thighs, buttocks, stomach, back, chest, arms, shoulders, neck, and face. Every muscle in your body is completely relaxed.

dence, and give you a greater sense of control over your race (to be discussed further in Chapter 6).

Ask yourself, "What do I need to do right now to perform my best?" This process focus can include paying attention to your technique or tactics. It might involve focusing on mental skills such as positive thinking or the psych-down strategies we're currently describing. You could shift your focus onto your breathing or muscle relaxation, which will take your mind off of the outcome and directly relax your body.

Keywords. Another focusing technique for lowering your intensity is to use intensity keywords. These words act as reminders of what you need to do with your intensity to perform well (see Intensity Keywords on page 69). Keywords are important in the midst of a race when you can get distracted by other competitors, the conditions, or your increasing fatigue and pain. Repeat psych-down keywords to yourself at various points in the race when your intensity starts to go up. We also recommend that you write one or two keywords on a piece of tape that you then put on a piece of your equipment, for example, on your handlebars. Looking at the written keyword acts as a further reminder to lower your intensity.

Music. Music is one of the most powerful tools you can use to control your intensity before races. We all know that music has a profound physical and emotional impact on us. Music has the ability to create happiness, sadness, inspiration, and pride. Music can also excite or relax us. Many world-class and professional athletes listen to music before they compete to help them reach their prime intensity.

Music is beneficial in several ways. It has a direct effect on you physically. Calming music slows your breathing and relaxes your muscles. Simply put, it makes you feel good. Mentally, it makes you feel positive and motivated. It also generates positive emotions, such as joy and contentment. Calming music also takes your mind off aspects of the race that may cause doubt or anxiety. The overall sensation of listening to relaxing music is a generalized sense of peace and well-being.

Smile. The last technique for lowering intensity is one of the strangest and most effective we've ever come across. A few years ago, Jim was working with a world-class athlete who was having a particularly bad workout. She was performing poorly and her coach was frustrated. She approached Jim during a break feeling angry, with her body in knots, and asked him what she could do. He didn't have an answer until an idea just popped into his head. He told her to smile. She said, "I don't want to smile." Once more, he told her to smile once more. She said she was not happy and didn't want to smile. He again told her to smile. This time, just to get him off her back, she did smile. He told her to hold the smile. During the next two minutes there was an amazing transformation. As she stood there with the smile on her face, the tension began to drain out of her body. Her breath-

INTENSITY KEYWORDS

Directions: A variety of intensity keywords have been provided below. In the space at the bottom, identify other intensity keywords that you can use.

Psych-Down	Psych-Up
Breathe	Go for it
Loose	Charge
Relax	Attack
Calm	Positive
Easy	Hustle
Trust	Commit

ing became slow and deep and her tense posture eased. In a short time, she was looking more relaxed and feeling better. She returned to her training, her workout improved, and she made progress during the remainder of the training session.

Her response was so dramatic that Jim wanted to learn how such a change could occur. When he returned to his office, he looked at the research related to smiling and learned two things. First, as we grow up, we become conditioned to the positive effects of smiling. In other words, we learn that when we smile, we're happy and life is good. Second, fascinating research that looked at the effects of smiling on our brain chemistry found that when we smile, it releases brain chemicals called endorphins, which have an actual physiologically relaxing effect.

You don't need to feel happy or good to smile. Smiling is a motor skill involving raising the corners of your mouth. Research has found that clenching a pencil in your teeth can make you feel happier because it forces your mouth into a smile. Smiling when you're nervous has the effect of relaxing your body and producing positive emotions. So next time you feel tense, smile!

> *On race day, remember to relax. You've done it all before. You're not asking your body to go out and do anything that it hasn't already done in training.*
>
> —Joe Friel

PSYCH-UP TECHNIQUES

Though letdowns in intensity are less common, they can also cause your level of performance to decline. Physically, you no longer have the blood flow, oxygen, and adrenaline necessary to maximize your strength and stamina. Mentally, you lose motivation and focus. Just like psych-down techniques when your intensity is too high, psych-up techniques can be used to raise your intensity when it drops.

Intense breathing. Just as deep breathing can reduce intensity, intense breathing can increase it. If you find your intensity dropping, several hard exhales can take your body and your mind to a more intense level. Intense breathing gets more oxygen into your system, increases blood flow and adrenaline, and generally energizes you. Mentally, intense breathing creates a more focused attitude and increases feelings of aggressiveness. It's a useful practice before a race, particularly at shorter distances.

Move your body. Intensity is, most basically, physiological activity. The most direct way to increase intensity is with physical action. In other words, move. Walk or run around, jump up and down, anything to get your body going. Moving your body increases heart rate, respiration, blood flow, and adrenaline. You'll shake off any lethargy you may feel and experience more energy, which is particularly important for shorter-distance races. You'll also feel more motivated, confident, and focused.

High-energy self-talk and body language. Letdown thoughts are one of the main causes of drops in intensity. Thinking to yourself, "I just don't have it today" or "I'm starting to bonk" will result in a decrease in your intensity. When this happens, your performance will decline. When you have these thoughts, replace them with high-energy self-talk, for example, "Keep attacking," "Finish strong," and "Stay pumped." This high-energy self-talk will raise your intensity and help you regain your motivation, confidence, and focus. Particularly late in races when you're tired and hurting, a constant internal monologue using high-energy self-talk can carry you through the tough parts and across the finish line. When you need to psych up, accompany your high-energy self-talk with similar body language, for example, pump your fist or slap your thigh. This combination of words and actions will increase your intensity and get you fired up.

Intensity keywords. Just as you can use keywords to lower intensity, they can also be used to counter letdowns and to psych yourself up (see page 69). Saying intensity keywords such as "Charge" and "Strong" with conviction and energy will raise your intensity, generate positive thoughts and emotions, and better enable you to perform well.

Music. The value of music has already been described above. Music can also be used to raise your intensity and get you psyched up and motivated. It can raise your heart rate, increase your respiration, and trigger the release of adrenaline. The overall sensation of listening to high-energy music is motivation, confidence, inspiration, and a generalized sense of excitement and energy.

TRIATHLETE SPOTLIGHT: STACY

Stacy was always a nervous wreck before races. At 47 years old, she had been doing triathlons with her husband, Ed, for almost a decade, but races never got any easier. She loved to train; giving her best effort, being around healthy people, and getting stronger was satisfying and fun for her. But starting a few days before every race, a knot would develop in her stomach and she'd have trouble sleeping.

Stacy came from a very competitive family in which her parents emphasized grades in schools and results in sports and put pressure on her and her siblings to be the best. Preperformance anxiety had become a regular—and uncomfortable—presence, whether she was taking a test in school, giving a presentation at work, or racing a triathlon. Her anxiety

(continued on next page)

(continued from previous page)

often hurt her performance, but, most importantly, she didn't enjoy herself as much as she would like. Her husband finally encouraged her to see a sport psychologist to find a solution.

Stacy always felt helpless to do anything about her anxiety, but she learned from the sport psychologist that she could do something to get rid of her nerves. Changing the way she thought about her race and actively relaxing her body could take the edge off her anxiety and make her feel a lot more comfortable. With her next race coming up, she focused on getting totally prepared. She spent extra time planning and executing her taper, getting her equipment in order, and organizing the trip with Ed. She noticed that by keeping busy with race-related preparations, she felt more in control and more relaxed. When she started to think about the race and feel nervous, she would take her mind off the outcome of the race and think about how she wanted to perform. She would also close her eyes, take a few deep breaths, smile, and think about how excited she was about the race.

Each evening after she got home from work, she put on some relaxing music, lay down, and followed the deep breathing and muscle relaxation exercises. She also imagined herself performing in different parts of the race; seeing herself more relaxed before the start and swimming, biking, and running well. After these sessions, she always felt better. In bed at night, she repeated the breathing and relaxation exercises, and found that she was falling asleep much more quickly. Ed even commented that she wasn't the ogre she typically was before races.

After feeling more relaxed leading up to the race, Stacy felt a little edgy on that morning, but much less nervous and uncomfortable than usual. During her early-morning preparations, she continued to focus on breathing deeply, staying relaxed, and getting her T1 organized. She also found that by talking to the many friends she saw, she didn't think about the race and actually enjoyed herself. Once the race got under way, she settled in and felt good. Periodically, she would begin to worry about how she would finish and feel anxiety coming on again. But she would ask herself, "What do I need to do now?" take a few deep breaths, and refocus on the moment at hand. Stacy had a great race, but, most importantly, she felt mostly relaxed and comfortable throughout and enjoyed herself much more.

CHAPTER

6 Focus

F ocus is one of the most misunderstood mental factors in sport. Most athletes think of focus as concentrating on one thing for a long time. But focusing in triathlon is much more complex. Triathlon requires you to focus on many things all at once over a time period ranging from one hour to seventeen hours. Your ability to focus effectively will often dictate your success in your race.

WHAT IS FOCUS?

Let's start with discussing a few key terms that will help you understand focus and how it affects your triathlon performance. Attentional field is everything inside of you (e.g., thoughts, emotions, and physical responses) and outside of you (e.g., sights and sounds) on which you could focus. Focus is the ability to attend to internal and external cues in your attentional field.

Prime focus involves focusing only on performance-relevant cues in your attentional field, focusing on cues that help you to perform well. Prime focus means having the ability to adjust your focus internally and externally as needed during the course of the race. It also involves being able to block out the many distractions that present themselves during a triathlon, such as flat tires, negative thoughts, and poor transitions.

Poor focus involves focusing on distractions in your attentional field, that is, focusing on cues that may hurt your performance. There are two types of distractions that can pull your attention away from a prime focus.

Interfering distractions are those that may directly hurt your performance, such as negative thoughts, anxiety, and concern over your result. Irrelevant distractions are those that simply distract you from an effective focus, but that don't directly interfere with your efforts, such as the scenic view during the bike, what you'll have for dinner after the race, or the project that is overdue at work. Achieving prime focus is challenging because prime focus cues and distractions can be the same thing. For example, during the swim, you need to focus on the swimmers around you, but if you get distracted by them, you won't pay attention to other important cues, such as your technique, pace, and course sighting.

▼

Ironman is all about focus. We all get to the start well trained. Successful athletes need to train themselves mentally to find their own emotional place to race from. For me, I need to feel happy to stay focused. Some people race well by gritting their teeth and getting angry at the world. For others, the dream of finishing is their means of staying motivated and focused.

—Lisa Bentley

Thinking vs. Focusing

There's a difference between thinking and focusing. This distinction influences not only your ability to concentrate on important aspects of triathlon, but it also affects your motivation, confidence, intensity, and emotions. Thinking is connected to your ego-investment in triathlon, that is, how important triathlon is to you. Thinking is judgmental and critical. If you make a mistake or perform poorly when you're in a thinking mode, it may hurt your confidence and cause you to feel badly about yourself as a triathlete. Thinking actually interferes with your ability to focus in a way that will help your performance and may cause it to deteriorate. You can tell whether you're thinking about triathlon by your emotional reactions when you're faced with challenging situations. If you're thinking, you're likely to react with strong emotions because these obstacles are blocking your path to your goals. You may feel any of a number of negative emotions ranging from annoyance and irritation to frustration, anger, and despair.

Focusing simply involves attending to internal or external cues. This process is objective and detached from judgment or evaluation. If you make a mistake on something you were focusing on, you're able to accept it and not be overly disappointed by the failure. In a focusing mode, you're able to use the failure as information to correct the problem and perform better in the future.

Focus Demands of Triathlon

Triathlon is a sport that places significant demands on your focus capabilities. Unlike other sports that have only a few important cues or that require only short spans of attention, triathlon has dozens of essential cues that must be attended to over the course of many hours. You can better adapt to these focus demands by recognizing the many cues that you focus on during a race. By understanding the diverse cues to which you have to attend, you will be more aware of them, see how they affect your performance, and can take steps to focus on performance-relevant cues and avoid distractions during training and races.

When you are simply paying attention to what is going on without thought, without judgment, you will be continually adjusting the few things you really do have control over in a race: speed, cadence, form, eating, drinking, and, of course, thought. Paying attention without thoughts gives you exactly what you need to race. It allows for immediate responses to the race as it unfolds without getting distracted by judgments.

—Mark Allen

Key focus areas of a triathlon include setting up T1 before the race and getting yourself physically, mentally, and logistically ready for the swim. During the swim, focus on your swim stroke and pace, other swimmers around you, and the course direction. At T1, putting the swim behind you, focus on making the physical and logistical transition to the bike, and settling into the first few miles of the bike. During the bike, focus on the road, course, and weather conditions, pace, body position, nutrition, other triathletes, and road hazards. As you enter T2, putting the bike behind you, focus on making the physical and logistical transition to the run, and getting comfortable during the first few miles. During the run, focus on your stride and pace, nutrition, and the course. As the race nears its end, focus on fatigue, pain management, and maintaining your form and pace to the finish line. Cues in triathlon can be categorized as either internal or external. "Focus Demands of Triathlon" (on page 76) suggests specific cues to focus on during a race.

FOCUS DEMANDS OF TRIATHLON

INTERNAL	EXTERNAL
Thoughts	Equipment
Emotions	Course (swim, bike, run)
Heart rate	Water temperature
Respiration	Water surface conditions
Muscles	Air temperature
Proprioception	Wind
Pre-race preparation	Terrain
Tactics	Road conditions
Technique (swim, bike, run)	Other competitors
Stroke	Road hazards/traffic
Cadence	Transitions
Stride	Distance
Body position	Speed
Nutrition	Time
Hydration	
Fatigue	
Pain	
Injuries	

Focus Style

One of the most important developments we've made in our work in recent years is in understanding the importance of identifying focus style. A focus style is a preference for paying attention to certain cues. You may be more comfortable focusing on some cues and avoiding or ignoring others. You have a dominant style that influences all aspects of your triathlon efforts. This dominant style will surface most noticeably when you're faced with challenging training or race conditions, such as cold water, a stiff headwind, or a hilly run course. The two types of focus styles are internal and external.

Internal focus style

Triathletes with an internal focus style perform best when they're totally and consistently focused on themselves during training or races. They keep their focus narrow, paying attention only to what they're doing.

These triathletes are easily distracted by activity in their immediate surroundings. If they broaden their focus and take their mind off themselves, for example, if they talk about nonsport topics with their training partner during a workout, they may become distracted and the quality of their training will decline. At races, triathletes with an internal focus style like to be left alone before the start and disengage from conversation with other competitors.

External focus style

Triathletes with an external focus style perform best when they broaden their focus and keep their minds off triathlon. They only focus on their training and race just prior to beginning a workout or the swim. These triathletes have a tendency to think too much and become negative and critical. This overly narrow focus causes them to lose confidence and experience overintensity. For these triathletes, it's essential that they take their focus away from triathlon except when actually training or racing. Even during races, triathletes with an external focus style can be seen talking with other competitors during the bike and run.

External focus style often runs counter to beliefs held by many triathletes and coaches. One may think that if triathletes aren't totally focused on their training or race, then they're not serious about the sport. Those with an external focus style, however, will perform best when they keep their focus wide, and don't think too much or become too serious.

I think the main thing for me is not ... to get too caught up in it. The main thing is to be casual and carefree and just go there and enjoy it and to have fun. For me, I don't like to necessarily be talking about triathlons all the time, so I like to have people around me where we're not always talking about the race coming up or the race we're at. We're talking about what's going on back home and stuff like that.

—Hunter Kemper,
2004 U.S. Olympic Triathlon Team

Identifying Your Focus Style

With an understanding of focus styles, you can now identify what your focus style is. Are you easily distracted and need to keep your mind on triathlon constantly to perform well? Or do you think too much and need to keep your mind off triathlon until it's time to train or race?

Recall past training and races when you've performed well. Were you totally focused on triathlon or were you keeping your mind off it? Also, recall past training and races when you've performed poorly. Were you thinking too much or were you distracted by things going on around you? Like most triathletes, a pattern will emerge in which you tend to perform best when you focus one way and you perform poorly when you focus another way.

Understanding your focus style is essential for managing it effectively. This process involves knowing how you focus best and actively focusing in a way that's consistent with your focus style. This ability to manage your focus style is most important in difficult training and race situations. Under pressure or when faced with adversity, you may revert to a focus style that will interfere with rather than help your performance. For example, if you're someone who performs best with an external focus style, you may find yourself turning your focus inward when things aren't going well. Thinking too much and becoming negative and critical may cause your performance to suffer.

When you start to lose your prime focus style under pressure, become aware that you're moving away from it and take steps to redirect your focus back to the style that works best for you. Continuing the previous example, when you realize that you're focusing too internally, actively direct your focus outward by taking your mind off triathlon.

Mag-Lite® Focus

The focus demands of triathlon require considerable flexibility in your focus capabilities. You must focus on many diverse cues during a triathlon, both internal and external, and a rigid focus style would limit your ability to focus on all the necessary cues. How well you can understand your focus style, be aware of helpful and harmful cues, and be flexible in your ability to focus will significantly affect your training and race performances.

Jim has developed a useful tool to help you understand your focus style and to develop focus control. A Mag-Lite® is a flashlight whose beam can be adjusted to illuminate a wide area or to brighten a narrow area. Your focus can be thought of as a Mag-Lite® beam you project that illuminates particular focus cues.

Triathletes with an internal focus style want to keep their Mag-Lite® beam narrow at all times, shining the focus light only on triathlon-related cues. If you have an internal focus style, your goal is to stay focused on necessary training or race cues and to block out unnecessary external distractions. To accomplish this, narrow your Mag-Lite® beam by keeping your eyes within the confines of the training or race setting and avoid talking to others. Focus on only important triathlon cues, for example, swim technique, a smooth pedal stroke, or an effective stride.

Triathletes with an external focus style want to widen their Mag-Lite® beam when they're not training or racing to take their minds off triathlon, then narrow their beam shortly before they begin a workout or a key part of a race. If you have an external focus style, your goal is to direct your focus off triathlon when it is not absolutely necessary. To do this, if you're riding or running along a part of the racecourse that isn't very demanding, widen your Mag-Lite® beam by looking around you or talking to other triathletes. This will keep you from shifting inward and thinking too much. Shortly before it's time to refocus on training or the race, narrow your Mag-Lite® beam, focusing specifically on something that will help you perform well.

There are also times when, regardless of your focus style, you'll need to narrow or widen your Mag-Lite® beam to adapt to the demands of the training or race situation. For example, as you begin the swim, widen your beam so you are aware of swimmers around you. When you are in T1 or T2, narrow your beam so you can focus completely on having a smooth transition.

Focus Control

Developing focus control is essential to ensuring that your focus style helps rather than hurts your performances. There are several steps in the focus-control process. Having identified your focus style and recognized internal and external cues that help and hurt your performances, you can now use focus-control strategies to adjust your focus internally and externally as needed.

The eyes have it. We obtain most of our information about the world through our eyes. The most direct way to control our Mag-Lite® beams is to control our eyes. You can think of your eyes as Mag-Lite® flashlights that you can adjust wide or narrow. If you want to minimize the external distractions during training and races, narrow your Mag-Lite® beam by keeping your eyes down and forward on the swim, bike, or run. If you're distracted by something, either look away or turn away from it. If you're not looking at something, it won't distract you.

Conversely, if you find that you're thinking too much, widen your Mag-Lite® beam by raising your eyes and looking around you, for example, see who's near you on the course. By looking around, you'll be distracted from your thoughts, clear your mind, and then you can narrow your Mag-Lite® beam back onto the current training or race situation.

Focus keywords. Developing focus keywords can be a simple way to maintain or regain your focus in training and races. Focus keywords are brief and descriptive reminders of what you need to focus on to perform well. Their value comes from your ability to refer to them quickly and easily when you need to focus on something that will help your performance. This accessibility is particularly important when you're struggling with distractions or late in a race when you're tired or in pain. In these situations you can get so wrapped up in the difficulties that you forget to focus on cues that will help you overcome the challenges. Repeat keywords to help you maintain your focus through a tough period. Keywords provide you with something to grab on to, to help you regain your focus when you become distracted. Focus keywords can be physical (e.g., easy breathing or long stride), technical (e.g., high elbow for swimming or head up for running), tactical (e.g., patience or finish strong), or mental (e.g., positive or attack).

Focus keywords are most effective when you create them in advance. Develop two or three keywords for each part of a triathlon. Pre-race keywords could include *relax, conserve,* or *breathe.* Swim examples might be *rhythm, long,* or *smooth.* Bike keywords could be *spin, patience,* or *fuel.* Run examples might be *form, even,* or *stride.* Transition keywords could be *settle down* or *one thing at a time.*

In the process of training with the utmost focus and determination of mind, body, and spirit, I was unconsciously locking myself away into a space that could only admit one result—Olympic selection. This created an incredible amount of pressure, which I mistook as a rising tide of passion, already near overflowing. [During my most important race] my body completely shut down. Nothing I could say or do would get it to perform the way I knew I had trained it to over the last eight months. I was choking. Yes, choking.
—Siri Lindley,
2000 ITU world champion

You strengthen the ability of keywords to help you focus by using them in training, particularly in situations when you get distracted. Practicing the use of focus keywords in training ingrains their use and value so when the same challenges arise in a race you can readily turn to them to help you maintain or regain your focus. Write your focus keywords on your equipment, for example, on your pre-race bag, handlebars, even on the back of your hand. These tangible reminders make doubly sure that you remember to focus on important things during races.

Relaxed body, focused mind. Research has shown that when your intensity moves above its prime level, focus narrows excessively and athletes can miss relevant cues. This finding is especially important in triathlon because there are so many things you must focus on to race well. Because of this relationship between intensity and focus, an effective way to improve your focus is to relax your body. Use the psych-down techniques we described in Chapter 5 to keep your body relaxed and protect your focus from becoming too narrow. Being relaxed will also remove common distractions associated with anxiety, for example, difficulty breathing, a racing heart, and muscle tension. Finally, feeling at ease will reduce distracting worries and allow you to focus on all of the things that are necessary for you to perform your best.

Outcome vs. process focus. Perhaps the greatest obstacle to prime focus is having an outcome focus during a race. Outcome focus involves focusing on the possible results of a race: winning, losing, rankings, or completion. Many triathletes believe that by focusing on the outcome, that is, on a certain result, they're more likely to achieve that outcome. Having an outcome focus, however, actually hurts performance and makes it less likely you'll achieve your goals. Every time you shift from a process focus to an outcome focus, your performance will decline. This drop in performance occurs for several reasons. First, you're no longer focusing on things that will help you execute well, for example, pace, exertion, and nutrition. Second, it causes your intensity to move away from prime intensity, either up because you start to get nervous or down because you think you already have the race in hand.

> *Take control of yourself and the race will follow your lead. Ninety miles into the bike [at the 1996 Hawaii Ironman®] I took control of my destiny—the race was no longer a disaster but a race that could still have incremental successes. Managing what I could control— my thoughts and feelings—allowed me to take command of my race.*
> —Dave Scott

The critical thing to remember is that the outcome occurs after the process is completed and the race is over. The outcome is totally unrelated to the process of the race. In fact, the result of an outcome focus is usually the exact opposite of the outcome you want, specifically, a great performance and achieving your race goals. The way to achieve the result you want is to focus on the process of the race, which involves, for example, technique, pace, pain management, and fueling. A valuable question to ask yourself to stay focused on the process is "What do I need to do now?" If you're answering this question, you'll be focusing on the things that will help you do your best. By focusing on the process, you're more likely to achieve your desired outcome.

Focus on what you can control. Only focus on things over which you have control. There are many aspects of a triathlon over which you can't exert any influence, such as your competitors, the weather, and course conditions. Focusing on these uncontrollable areas detracts from your efforts to perform your best. There's only one thing that you can control in your triathlon training and racing, and that is yourself, for example, your attitude, thoughts, emotions, intensity, effort, technique, tactics, and nutrition. If you focus on those areas that you can control, you'll be sure that you're doing everything you can to achieve your goals.

Once in the race, it seems that being present and aware of what is going on is more important. I constantly think as I am racing, "How do I feel, what do I need, is my pace OK?" By going through this over and over, I am being present and accountable for everything that is going on with my body.

—Heather Fuhr

Four Ps. We have a general rule you can follow that will help you identify what areas to focus on in triathlon. We call them the four Ps. The first P is *positive*. Focus on positive things that will help your performance and avoid negative things that will hurt it. The second P is *process*. As we've just explained, focus on what you need to do during the race, not on what might happen at the end of the race. The third P is *present*. You should focus on what you can do at the present moment of the race rather than on the past (which can't be controlled) or the future (which can only be controlled by influencing the present). The last P is *progress*. Triathletes often compare themselves with other triathletes when their focus should be on their own improvement. What's important is that you see yourself progressing toward the goals you want to achieve.

TRIATHLETE SPOTLIGHT: ZACH

Zach, a 14-year-old, had wanted to do triathlons since he saw Simon Whitfield win the sport's first gold medal at the 2000 Olympic Games in Sydney. He had trained hard the last three years and had progressed steadily through the junior ranks to the point where he was now in the top twenty in his age group nationally. But, ever since starting in triathlon, Zach felt he was holding himself back. He had trouble focusing for extended periods of time, and his distractibility had cost him better results in several races. For example, he would get distracted in transitions with all of the activity going on around him and with so many things to do. He would either take too much time getting his act together or he would forget something, such as gels or his sunglasses. During the bike and the run, his mind would wander and his pace would unconsciously slow. He had the same focusing problem in school, and his parents had him tested for ADD. The results indicated a mild attentional impairment that his doctor said could affect him in his triathlons. The exercises his doctor gave him helped him in school, but didn't translate well to triathlon.

After reading an article by a sport psychologist in one of the tri-mags, Zach told his parents that he wanted to see one to help him focus better in races. In their first session, the sport psychologist, Dr. R., said that focusing problems were common among triathletes and there were some specific techniques Zach could use to help him maintain his focus throughout a race. The first thing Dr. R. suggested was for Zach to lay out his transition area in a very organized and consistent way. She then told him to create the transition layout at home and practice it until he could do it without thinking. Dr. R. then recommended that, in the last 100 yards of the swim and the last half mile of the bike, he shift his focus to his transition and briefly review what he would need to do. To help him focus better, she told Zach that as soon as he got out of the water, he should focus on taking slow, deep breaths to relax his body and direct his focus to his transition area. He could do the same thing in the last quarter mile of the bike before T2. Zach should also narrow his Mag-Lite® beam as soon as he enters the T1 and T2, keeping his eyes down and forward, only focusing on his transition area.

Dr. R. told Zach that the best way to maintain focus during races was to practice that focus in training. She suggested that he come up with keywords he could say to himself that would remind him of what to focus

(continued on next page)

(continued from previous page)

on. For example, during the bike, Zach would lose his focus and his cadence would drop, so he came up with "spin fast" as keywords. He decided to write these words on a piece of tape that he placed on his handlebars. During the run, Zach would begin to tire and focus too much on his discomfort, so he would slow down. To counter this tendency, he chose "long and strong" as his keywords to remind him to keep his stride long and his pace strong.

After working on Dr. R.'s recommendations for six weeks, Zach felt much more focused and confident in himself. During the race, he had fewer distractions and, when he lost focus, he was able to regain it quickly by repeating his keywords. And he had a great race, finishing in the top five in a national event for the first time. He also noticed that he was more focused in school, which was reflected in better grades in his classes.

C H A P T E R

7 Emotions

When people reflect on triathlon, many think about the profound physical challenges triathletes face in training and races. Yet, based on our own triathlon experience and feedback from the many triathletes with whom we have worked, the physical side of triathlon, though certainly arduous, is not the most demanding. The consensus is that the emotional aspects of triathlon are the most taxing. During the course of your training and races you will experience the entire spectrum of emotions. You may feel exhilaration, pride, fulfillment, and contentment. You may also feel fear, frustration, disappointment, and despair. Not only will you experience all of these emotions, but you may feel them regularly, unpredictably, and with increasing force as you move to longer races.

The highs and lows of emotion are a normal and healthy part of triathlon. In fact, emotions may be why you participate in the sport. Triathlon causes you to feel deeply, perhaps more deeply than you feel in other parts of your life. And when you feel emotions with such acuteness and power, you feel alive and vital. The downside to feeling emotions so strongly is that you don't just feel the positive emotions. Emotions are two sides of the same coin so you must also be willing to feel the so-called bad emotions. Your goal is not to avoid the negative emotions—you can't. Rather, you want to accept the negative emotions, figure out what's causing them, resolve them, and replace them with positive emotions.

VALUE OF EMOTIONS

The emotions you experience can tell you a lot about yourself physically. Your emotions are a valuable gauge of your training. They are perhaps the best measure of whether you've struck the proper balance among volume, intensity, and recovery in your training. When you have that balance, you're happy, excited, and motivated. When you've lost that balance, you're frustrated, irritable, and depressed, and your body is telling you that changes are needed.

Because of the constant and intense demands that you place on your body during triathlon training, you will experience considerable ups and downs physically, from feeling thoroughly energized to completely spent. Your emotions will parallel how you feel physically and, because of these fluctuations, you may be riding an emotional roller coaster during your triathlon season. This ride really hit home for Steve, a midpack age grouper who was training for his first half-Ironman race. In his first year of triathlon, during which he raced a number of sprint and Olympic-distance events, he had gone through an extended period of what we call the "tri-high," in which he was in a constant state of excitement about his training and races. He went to bed jazzed and woke up psyched to hit the pool, road, and track. And his happiness permeated every part of his life.

But in his second season, his ride got a bit bumpy. Early in the year, following a three-week high-volume, high-intensity training block, he found that he was one unhappy guy—cranky, depressed, and just plain not enjoying life. He had no joy in his training and was questioning the time and energy he was devoting to triathlon. Steve had a recovery week scheduled so he backed off his training. In a few days, he started to get his good feelings back and, by the end of the week, he was excited about triathlon again. Steve found this pattern continued throughout his season and he learned what it meant and how to deal with it.

Your emotions can tell you about your training intensity and your level of general life stress. Negative emotions, such as frustration, anger, and melancholy, are more likely to arise when your intensity is too high. When you're stressed, you're more sensitive to negative emotions and more likely to feel them more acutely. You're also likely to feel negative emotions in your training and racing if you're experiencing stress away from triathlon. Stress in your personal, social, or professional life can make you more vulnerable to negative emotions you experience in the sport.

A result of continued high-intensity training and life stress is a decline in the effectiveness of your immune system. If your immune system can't adequately manage your training demands, your body may break down. You may feel ongoing fatigue, fail to get enough sleep, and lack motivation and energy to train. You may get sick and not be able to shake it off. You may sustain minor injuries that don't seem to heal. In each of these cases you will feel negative emotions more frequently and more strongly.

Your emotions can be a measure of your nutritional intake in training and races. There is a relationship between inadequate nutrition and negative emotions. Particularly in longer races, a downward shift in emotions can signal a nutritional crisis, that is, a drop in blood sugar, insufficient calories, or dehydration. Stay conscious of this connection and respond promptly to prevent further emotional and nutritional deterioration. An essential lesson to learn is that, even when you feel yourself in an inescapable pit of despair, you can bring yourself back from declining emotions and a nutritional deficit and return to positive emotions and optimal energy by refueling immediately.

The common theme throughout this discussion is the significant relationship between your physiology (i.e., intensity, stress, fatigue, illness, injury, nutrition) and your emotions. If you're physically stable, your emotions will be up. If your body is struggling physically in some way, your emotions may be down. Using your emotions as a litmus test to how you're doing physically can help you get yourself physically back on track and relieve any negative emotions you're feeling.

Causes of Negative Emotions in Training and Races

Emotions that can arise in triathlon (and life) come from past experiences in the form of beliefs you hold about yourself and your attitude toward your achievement efforts, such as sports participation. Negative emotions associated with these beliefs are commonly known as the "baggage" people carry from their upbringings, for example, fear of failure and pre-race anxiety. This baggage, which may have served a purpose when you were a child, can cause you to respond to present situations in ways that go against your best interests.

Negative emotions can also be provoked by unforeseen or unfortunate occurrences in your training and races. One of the great lessons triathletes learn is from Murphy's Law: Whatever can go wrong will go wrong at the worst possible moment. Murphy's Law creates obstacles, setbacks, and just plain bad luck that cause many negative emotions. You feel frustration when you get a flat or lose a water bottle from its cage. Rough water, unseasonably hot weather, or a stiff headwind can cause feelings of helplessness and despair. You feel anger when a group of riders pass you drafting in a no-drafting race. You feel disappointment when you bonk in the middle of the run. You feel fear when faced with an injury. Not showing progress in your training, having a bad race, or failing to perform up to your expectations can all cause you to feel any of these negative emotions. All of these events share two common elements that lie at the heart of what causes the negative emotions: You may feel that the path to your goals is being blocked and that you don't believe you have control over removing the obstacle.

Emotions can unwittingly become habits that cause you to automatically respond with a certain negative reaction to a particular circumstance even when that emotional response does more harm than good. For example, Susan had flats in three consecutive races resulting in a DNF and two poor finishes. She was devastated by these unfortunate experiences and developed a belief that she was cursed. In subsequent races, she was terrified of getting a flat whenever the road got rough. She became cautious, believing that hitting uneven pavement at a higher speed would cause a blowout. Because of her tentative riding, she never performed up to her expectations. When she flatted in a race a few months later, she was so upset that she couldn't change her own tire and waited thirty minutes for the support van to change it for her.

Ultimately, emotions are a natural reaction to the normal ups and downs of life. When life is going well, you feel happy, contented, and excited. When life is going poorly, you feel frustrated, disappointed, and sad. When life is just going, you feel bored and blasé. Never resist your emotions, but rather allow yourself to experience them, understand them, and, if they are unpleasant, ride them out or try to change them.

Effects of Emotions on Triathletes

Negative emotions hurt performance both physically and mentally. Negative emotions cause you to lose your prime intensity. With frustration and anger, your intensity may go up and lead to muscle tension and breathing difficulties. It may sap your energy and cause you to tire quickly. When you experience disappointment and despair, your intensity drops sharply and you no longer have the physiological capabilities (i.e., respiration, blood flow, and adrenaline) necessary to perform well. Positive emotions also have a significant impact on your physiology. When you're contented, your body is calm and relaxed. When you're excited, your body is energized. Positive emotions aid in keeping you focused and motivated on your execution and goals.

Negative emotions also hurt you mentally. Fundamentally, negative emotions are a response to the perceived threat that you will fail to achieve your goals. Your emotions are telling you that, deep down, you're not confident that you can be successful. Your confidence will decline and you may feel doubt and uncertainty. Also, because negative emotions are so strong, you may have difficulty focusing on what will help you perform well. Negative emotions can hurt your motivation to train and compete because they take the enjoyment out of your triathlon experiences. What makes the relationship among these mental factors so challenging is that they can feed on one another, creating a vicious cycle of decline in one or more of them. For example, a loss of confidence and increased intensity can trigger negative emotions that, in turn, hurt the other mental areas.

Positive emotions offer many mental benefits. Positive emotions motivate you to pursue your goals because they reward your efforts with good feelings. They foster positive thinking, which builds confidence. Positive emotions encourage you to stay focused by removing the negative aspects of your performance that cause distractions. And they reduce the pain you experience by releasing neurochemicals that act as an anesthetic (see Chapter 8 for more on the relationship between emotions and pain).

THREAT VS. CHALLENGE

A simple distinction between threat and challenge appears to lie at the heart of your emotional reactions. Emotional threat can arise when you become overly invested in triathlon. In essence, your self-esteem—how you feel about yourself as a person—becomes overly connected to how you perform in training and races. Triathlon becomes a threat when you enter the "too zone" that we described in Chapter 1. Emotional threat is often associated with pressure that is self-imposed or forced on you by others, such as family, friends, or training partners. Every time you train or race, your self-esteem is on the line. You're driven to avoid failure because you perceive it as a direct attack on your self-worth as a person. With this belief, it's easy to see why triathlon can be emotionally threatening.

Emotional threat can cause a fight-or-flight reaction, which is aimed at relieving the threat. The fight response is expressed when you develop an extreme motivation to train. You may push yourself unmercifully, trying to reach a level of fitness that will ensure success and reduce the emotional threat, but you push so hard that you may overtrain, get injured, or burn out. This reaction may also cause you to go out in a race at a pace that you can't sustain, causing you to bonk and to fail to achieve your race goals. This fight response, rather than alleviating the emotional threat, can cause the very thing—failure—that is so threatening to you in the first place.

The flight response can lead to a loss of motivation to train and race. If you're not in good physical condition because you didn't train, expectations for race success will be low. In races where the threat of failure is so immediate and strong, this response may lead you to slow down or drop out when you're doing poorly. By being out of shape, quitting, or slowing down, you're able to protect your self-esteem because you have an excuse for why you failed.

In contrast, emotional challenge is associated with caring deeply about triathlon, but not entering into the "too zone." You enjoy the process of triathlon—the training, the camaraderie, the races—regardless of how you do. You gain pleasure out of all aspects of your training and see races as an opportunity to see what you are capable of. Triathlon, when seen as an emotional challenge, is an experience that you relish and seek out. You strive to give your best effort and accept when you don't perform up to your expectations. Emotional challenge is expressed in the strong desire to push yourself beyond your perceived limits, to achieve your goals, and to grow as a triathlete and person. Importantly, you have triathlon in perspective and maintain a healthy balance of triathlon and other parts of your life. Emotional challenge is highly motivating, to the point where you love being faced with the challenge that triathlon presents.

> *I vividly remember the '96 Ironman, trying not to dwell on my extraordinarily slow swim and searching for renewed confidence.... Watching Thomas Hellriegel and Peter Reid fly by me at the airport diluted my momentum further. After wrestling with several hours of negative thoughts, I finally turned my destructive pattern into a positive challenge. The race was no longer a disaster, but a race in which I could still have incremental successes.*
>
> —Dave Scott

DEVELOPING EMOTIONAL MASTERY

How we respond to emotional situations is at least partially hardwired into us at birth. Some of us are more sensitive, others more volatile, still others more stoic. At the same time, "genetics is not destiny"; in other words, you don't have to be at the mercy of your emotions. Some people, *emotional victims*, believe that they have little control over their emotions. If their emotions hurt them, they believe they just have to accept it because they can't do anything about it. However, you're capable of gaining control of your emotions and becoming an *emotional master*.

Steps to Emotional Mastery

Changing your emotions is a significant mental challenge because emotions are so deeply ingrained due to genetics and past experiences. To change emotions, you have to start with believing that change is possible. Emotions are a simple, but not easy, choice. If you have the option to feel badly and perform poorly or feel good and perform well, you will certainly choose the latter option. However, past emotional baggage and old emotional habits can lead you to respond emotionally in the present in ways that are not in your best interests. The choice comes with your awareness of when old emotional baggage and habits arise, and then choosing a positive emotional response that will lead to good feelings and a successful performance.

Changing your emotions might require you to examine your emotional baggage. If the emotions are strong and they significantly interfere with not only your triathlon participation, but many aspects of your life, you might consider seeking help from a qualified counselor or psychologist. Such guidance can assist you in better understanding and letting go of your baggage and learning new emotional responses that will better serve you in triathlon and life.

Emotional mastery begins with recognizing the negative emotional reactions that hurt your triathlon efforts. When you start to feel negative emotions in training and races, be aware of what emotions you're feeling, for instance, frustration, anger, or despair. Identify which situations cause them, for example, when a rider who you thought you were stronger than passes you on a climb. Consider what the underlying cause of the emotions is, such as feeling weak or inadequate.

Emotions that interfere with performance are often due to poor emotional habits that can be retrained, much as you retrain poor swimming, cycling, or running techniques. To continue the process of emotional mastery in training and races, specify alternative emotional reactions to situations that commonly trigger negative emotions. For example, instead of yelling, "I am so slow" and feeling despair when you get dropped during a ride, say, "Focus and be strong" and produce feelings of pride in your efforts and inspiration in knowing you're working toward your goals. This positive emotional response will help you let go of the initial negative emotions, motivate you to maintain your effort and intensity, generate positive emotions that will give you more confidence, and allow you to focus on what will help you raise the level of your performance.

Gaining emotional mastery and instilling positive emotional reactions takes time to solidify because your negative emotional habits may be well ingrained. With practice, and the realization that you feel and perform better with positive emotional responses, you will in time retrain your emotions into a positive emotional skill that will help you achieve your goals.

THREE EMOTIONAL CHALLENGES

You will experience many different emotions during triathlon training and races: inspiration, irritation, pride, disappointment, joy, and sadness. Some feel good, others feel lousy. Some help you go fast, others feel like anchors tied around your waist. There are three negative emotions, however, that are the most difficult to overcome and that will not only keep you from achieving your competitive goals, but will also suck the joy out of your triathlon efforts: fear, frustration, and despair.

I finally came to the realization that training wasn't just about the physical—swimming, cycling, and running; it was practicing the mental stuff too. And probably the most important mental aspect is dealing with the things you're afraid of.

—Paul Huddle

Fear

Triathlon can be a scary sport. It presents triathletes with many fear-provoking experiences with potentially harmful immediate and long-term consequences. These fears are a double-edged sword. One edge of the sword is the very real fears of physical harm and death, most often associated with swimming and cycling, as well as fear of injury, fear of pain, and psychological fears, such as fear of failure. The other edge of the sword is that these dangers can be what make triathlon so challenging, exciting, and fulfilling. But, despite this exhilaration, fear is most often an uncomfortable and physically and emotionally debilitating experience that hurts your performances and detracts from your triathlon experience. By understanding and actively combating your fear, you'll be in a better position to perform your best and enjoy your training and race efforts.

Fear of physical harm or death

Two of the three disciplines in triathlon—swimming and cycling—can be potentially dangerous. Open-water swimming removes the security of pool walls, shallowness, warm water, lifeguards, and clear water, and can be a source of profound fear for many triathletes, particularly newbies or those who don't have an extensive background in swimming. When swimming in the ocean is added to the mix, with its murkiness and the real or imagined danger of shark attacks, fear can be crippling. The added threat of mass starts that are used in many races adds to the fear quotient. Swim starts usually have swimmers packed in tightly who are often unable or unwilling to give ground. This situation leads to considerable contact, rough water, difficulty sighting, and a fear of drowning. The potential for fear and panic is real.

I've always been afraid of the crosswinds, and that's not a good way to ride your bike.

—Lori Bowden

Cycling presents a different danger and cause for fear. Every time you go for a ride, you are putting yourself in harm's way. Most cyclists know or have heard about someone who either crashed or was hit by a car and sustained a serious injury or who died from a cycling accident. What makes this fear so difficult is that you don't always have control over the danger and it often arises unexpectedly, for example, a pothole in the road or a car backing out of a driveway. Additionally, cars and trucks aren't always accommodating to bicycles and some drivers are downright hostile.

Fear of injury

Triathlon places significant demands on your body and these demands increase as the race distances get longer and the frequency, duration, and intensity of training builds. It's rare for a triathlete not to sustain an injury due to overuse, improper technique, or inadequate recovery. The occurrence of injuries, particularly when they are serious—for example, a torn rotator cuff from swimming, or recurrent, such as a nagging hamstring pull from speed work on the track—can cause you to fear continuing your training efforts and discourage you from moving up to longer races. These fears can also reduce your motivation to train and limit the intensity you put into your training.

Fear of pain

Perhaps the most immediate fear triathletes face is the fear of pain from exertion. Pain experienced during training and races is a normal part of triathlon, and all triathletes know they will feel it at some point. Some pain is one reason people do triathlons. It offers meaning, satisfaction, and affirmation of your efforts. Most people will tell you that the more they suffer, the more rewarding it was. But there is a line where the pain isn't worth it, and it is crossing the line that triathletes fear. This fear may cause you to hold back early in a race out of worry that you won't have enough energy and will suffer too much at the end. This fear, paradoxically enough, will also cause you to feel more pain when it does arrive (more on this issue in Chapter 8). Fear of pain arises most often among tri-newbies who have less familiarity with training and race pain, and who have fewer coping skills to manage the pain they experience.

> *Fear of pain—fear of discomfort. Sometimes I didn't think that the fear would go away, though now I realize I might have been happier going through it. Sometimes I crossed the finish line more in one piece than I would have wanted and lamenting I didn't throw down like I would have liked.*
>
> —Paul Huddle

Fear of failure

In addition to fears of bodily injury, psychological fears can interfere with you enjoying your triathlon participation and achieving your goals. Common among these fears is the fear of failure that can arise when you become overly invested in your triathlon efforts. Fear of failure is commonly thought of as a belief that failure will result in some type of bad consequence, for example, disappointing others, losing respect, feeling shame and embarrassment, or devaluing oneself. Fear of failure is so palatable because people connect their results with whether they will be loved and valued by themselves or others. In other words, how they feel about themselves is based on whether they succeed or fail to live up to their expectations. Most people are motivated to succeed and to gain affirmation from themselves and praise from others. But those who fear failure are often driven to avoid failure and the criticism and negative impressions that they believe will come with it. Their self-esteem is based on their ability to avoid failure and gain self-love by achieving success. Fear of failure is a potent and unhealthy influence on people and has been associated with many psychological difficulties including low self-esteem, eating disorders, drug abuse, depression, anxiety, and suicide.

> *Fear is probably the thing that limits performance more than anything—the fear of not doing well, of what people will say. You've got to acknowledge those fears, then release them.*
>
> —Mark Allen

Psychological Impact of Fear

Fear can be a powerful psychological obstacle to achieving your triathlon goals. Regardless of the source of your fear, it may create a cascade of deficits in psychological areas that are essential for triathlon success. Fear reduces your motivation to train and race because doing so is physically and psychologically uncomfortable. Fear hurts your confidence because, inherent in any fear is the belief that some form of harm—whether physical or mental—will come from your efforts. This loss of motivation and confidence may cause you to become cautious and tentative, and prevent you from fully committing yourself to your efforts. Fear also cripples your ability to focus. The emotional and physical experiences of fear are so strong that it is difficult to focus on things that will help your performance. Fear also strangles any enjoyment you may have in your triathlon participation.

Physical Impact of Fear

Fear expresses itself profoundly in the physical symptoms you feel, including anxiety, muscle tension, shallow breathing, and loss of coordination. These physical sensations individually and collectively create tremendous discomfort. The physical indications of fear can burn unnecessary energy, interfere with effective movement, and reduce cardiovascular efficiency.

The cumulative physical symptoms of fear interfere with your ability to perform your best.

Mastering Fear

Fear is an essential human emotion that protects you when your physical well-being is threatened. Unfortunately, fear can also arise in situations where it is neither required nor helpful. People often think of courage as the absence of fear, but true courage is being able to perform in the face of fear. Your goal when you experience fear is not to banish it thoroughly, but rather to master the fear and remove it as an obstacle to your goals.

Fears come in all shapes and sizes. A recent survey we conducted with the Golden Gate Triathlon Club (GGTC) in San Francisco offered interesting insights into common fears among triathletes. Some fears are rational; in other words, there is something that is worthy of fear, for example, being afraid of crashing during a high-speed descent on your bike. Other fears are entirely irrational, such as worry about a shark attack in a freshwater lake (this fear is more common than you might think). Some fears have to do with physical injury or death, for example, twisting an ankle during a trail run or drowning during a swim. Other fears have to do with your race performances, such as getting a flat and having to drop out of a race or bonking on the run. Still other fears are related to psychological injury, such as failing to achieve a race goal and feeling like a failure.

However realistic or farfetched your fears, they are as real as you believe them to be. Fears also don't just go away on their own. They can be persistent and become ingrained into your thinking and emotions. To stop fears, you have to face them, deal with them, and put them behind you. Being free of fears will liberate you to push yourself to your limits, achieve your goals, and enjoy your triathlon experiences.

Understand your fear. The first step to mastering your fear is to understand what your fear is. Is the cause of your fear obvious, such as riding on a narrow shoulder of a road with considerable traffic? Or is the source of your fear less clear, for example, feeling pre-swim fear that you attribute to the cold water but is actually caused by worry about failing to achieve your goals? It's important to understand the precise cause of the fear to address and relieve it.

Part of understanding your fear is becoming familiar with it. In what situation does it arise? What thoughts are associated with the fear? How does the fear make your body feel? What lessens your fear? Having a clear understanding of your fear enables you to directly address its cause and, as a result, relieve it as quickly and easily as possible.

Gain perspective of your fear. The GGTC survey we conducted showed widespread agreement on the fears we describe in this section. If you're experiencing fear in a triathlon situation, the chances are you're not alone. The fears we just discussed are likely felt by many triathletes around you. This shared experience tells you that the fear you're feeling is normal. Recognizing that your fear is felt by others will help keep it in perspective and prevent the fear from consuming you. Part of gaining perspective on fear involves the realization that the fear doesn't have to cripple you and that you have the power to master the fear. Talking to others about your fear can help you normalize your fear and give you insights into how they deal with their fears.

Master your fear. Rational fears are best resolved by finding a solution to the cause of the fear. By gaining relevant information, experience, and skills, you may alleviate the source of the fear. Or by changing the situation that causes the fear, you can remove the source of the fear and prevent the fear from arising. For example, a fear of a mass swim start is common among triathletes because of the close quarters, frantic pace, flailing bodies, and rough water. This fear can be relieved in several ways. You can gain experience and comfort with mass starts by creating the feeling of a mass start during open-water practice swims with your training buddies and becoming more skilled at staying relaxed, maintaining your swim stroke, and "Tarzan" swimming (head out of the water) to ensure that you're able to see, breathe, and navigate more readily. You can avoid the jostling that causes your fear by starting at the back of the pack and allowing the large pack to thin out in the first part of the swim. You can also reframe the situation from being fearful to being excited in anticipation of the start of the race. Another example, the fear of a high-speed descent on your bike, can be relieved in several ways as well. Take bike-handling classes that will improve your cycling skills and give you more confidence in your descents. Gain more experience and comfort by doing a great deal of descending on your training rides. An alternative way to relieve your fear is to simply slow down on the descents, realizing that triathlons are rarely won or lost on the downhills of the bike.

Mastering irrational fears involves a different approach. Because there is no solution to irrational fears, you can't solve the fear or readily change the situation that causes the fear. Instead, you have to counter the irrational beliefs that cause the fear, in other words, be rational with your irrationality. Returning to the example of shark attacks in freshwater lakes, remind yourself that there are no sharks in lakes, and even if one were released into a lake, it would die quickly because it needs salt water to survive. For good measure, you can do an Internet search to confirm that there has never been a shark attack in a lake. You can also draw on your own experiences and that of your friends swimming in lakes and recognize that you have never seen or heard of a shark in a lake. Even with this rational debunking, your irrational fears may linger. When the fear pops up, accept it as normal, decide to put it out of your mind, and focus on tangible aspects of your swim.

Regardless of whether your fears are rational or irrational, you can use several practical techniques to help you overcome the fears. Positive thinking that focuses on your strengths and your ability to overcome your fears will gird you against the force of those fears. You can resist being consumed by the fear by focusing on things that will help you deal with the fear; for example, you can focus on sighting off the buoys or optimal technique on the bike during high-speed descents. If you're focused on the process, you won't be focusing on the fear.

For seven years I faced the irrevocable, implacable force of Dave Scott in Hawaii. It was a supreme test to go there thinking I was deserving and prepared to win. When every time . . . I could see I was in some way not ready, physically, emotionally, spiritually, mentally. I was basically intimidated by the race, the conditions, and Dave. For a long time I didn't know how to deal with Hawaii. It was a very powerful place, and I needed to find a way to gain strength from its intensity instead of becoming scared by it. I was on the verge of giving up and never coming back. I had to have the courage to go through the race and win.

—Mark Allen

Because fears express themselves physically in terms of muscle tension, increased heart rate, and shallow breathing, you can also reduce your fear by using deep breathing and muscle relaxation. Creating a physical state that counters the feelings of fear will cause you to feel less fear. This strategy has the added benefit of distracting you from the fear, helping you focus on something that actually lessens your fear, and increasing your sense of control over your fear. In cases where the fear is irrational or can cause little real harm, a great way to get over your fear is to just accept it and get on with what you're doing. We've found that the most fear-provoking part of triathlon is just thinking about your fears. Once you get into it, it's rarely as bad you as you had imagined. Finally, don't expect your fear to disappear overnight. Be patient, work on overcoming your fear, and as you gain experience, confidence, and comfort, you'll often find that the fear fades.

FRUSTRATION

Frustration is at the heart of many negative emotional reactions you experience in triathlon. Frustration, in its most basic form, is the emotion you feel when your efforts toward your goals are thwarted. For example, if your goal is to maintain a comfortable and consistent pace early in the race and pass competitors on the run, then you may get frustrated if you're unable to maintain a good rhythm on the swim and bike, and you're getting passed on the run.

Frustration can initially be motivating because it pushes you to find ways to remove the obstacles to your goal. But if you're unable to turn the race around, then the initial frustration may become more persistent and could morph into anger. Anger can also be useful because you may become even more motivated to clear the path to your goals. Your intensity may shoot up and your pace may increase, which can be beneficial if the race is short or you're near the finish. But if you're in a longer race or you get angry early, your anger may hurt you. You may not be able to think or focus clearly, or figure out how to remove the obstacles that caused the initial frustration. Your anger may also burn fuel unnecessarily and cause you to run out of gas before the finish. If you are still unable to clear the obstacles to your goals, you may lapse into despair, which we discuss on page 102.

Attitude toward Frustration

Adversity is a normal and inevitable part of triathlon. Rare is the race in which nothing goes awry. Frustration often arises in the face of this adversity, for example, jostling at the start of the swim, a poor transition, or a stiff headwind. If everyone faces adversity in a triathlon, what separates those who get frustrated and have poor races from those who don't is how you react to the adversity. The triathletes who are most successful are those who respond best to the challenges with which they are faced.

Responding positively to frustration can prevent other stronger and more harmful negative emotions from arising. Your goal is to react positively to the first signs of frustration. This reaction starts with developing a positive attitude toward common causes of frustration in triathlon, such as a slow start, poor transitions, mechanical failures, inclement weather, or bad course conditions. Accept that you will have problems and days when things just don't go your way. Also recognize that you aren't the only one who has to deal with these problems. Overcoming adversity on a challenging day can still give you a satisfying race and teach you valuable lessons you can use in the future, for example, the benefits of staying positive, motivated, relaxed, and focused.

> We should pray for it, heat, wind, chop. We should know how to deal with it and look for it to help us. A lot of other people aren't prepared for it. But if we are, we're one up on them. The conditions should be an observation, not a complaint. You notice it but don't let it bother you. If you've trained in adversity this will come naturally.
>
> —Paul Huddle

Recognizing Frustration

With this attitude toward frustration in place, you're in a position to take practical steps to counter the frustration you will periodically experience. First, learn to identify the situations in which frustration usually arises. Perhaps it occurs during the swim because you have the least confidence in this event. Maybe it's when you're riding on a rolling course that doesn't allow you to establish a rhythm. Or perhaps you get frustrated because you never seem to have a strong run finish.

If you've gotten frustrated under certain circumstances in previous races, you're likely to get frustrated in a similar situation in future races. If you can recognize the frustration coming on, you can do something to either avoid it before it comes up or let it go when it does. Having realized that frustration may be just around the corner, you can find a solution to the problem that causes the frustration in the first place. For example, if you get frustrated during a mass swim start, you can master your frustration by swimming to clear water so you're not bumped around. If you start to get frustrated riding into a headwind, remind yourself that everyone has to deal with the headwind, stay relaxed, and adjust your effort accordingly.

When faced with adversity and the possibility of having negative emotions overwhelm you, realize that you have the opportunity to be an emotional master rather than an emotional victim. As an emotional master, you can choose how you will react to how you're doing in training and races. How quickly you make the choice in response to frustration will determine how long you continue to feel and perform poorly. The sooner you make the right choice, the sooner you can feel better and raise your performance.

Mastering Frustration

To reduce the effects of frustration when it arises, shift your thinking in a more positive direction. Remind yourself of how well you've trained and how prepared you are. Because frustration can be caused by obstacles to your goals, focus on the process of the race. Ask yourself, "What can I do to deal with this situation?" If you're focusing on everything over which you have control, you'll be in a better position to find a solution to the cause of the frustration.

We're sure you've been in this situation before. You start to get frustrated about something and someone tells you, "Relax. Take it easy." That response may make you more frustrated because if it was that easy, you would already have relaxed and taken it easy, but it's actually great advice. A powerful way to resist frustration is to create a physical state that counters your frustration. One way you know you're experiencing emotion is by the physical changes that occur. You notice you're frustrated when your heart rate increases, your breathing becomes shallow, your adrenaline flows, and your muscles tense. If you can reduce the bodily sensations associated with frustration, you may not feel your frustration as strongly.

The next time you feel yourself getting frustrated, focus on your body and take steps to relax. Referring to the psych-down techniques we describe in Chapter 5, you can use deep breathing, muscle relaxation, calming keywords, and smiling to help you gain a more relaxed physical state. With all of these strategies, you will be mentally, physically, and emotionally better equipped to overcome your frustration and continue on your path to your goals.

DESPAIR

Despair is the most difficult emotion to deal with because it carries feelings of finality and hopelessness. When you feel despair, you've lost confidence in your ability to continue. Your motivation to work disappears. All of the physical attributes that enabled you to maintain your efforts, including heart rate, respiration, and blood flow, can decline dramatically. When you experience despair, you slow your pace and give up mentally. Despair is so emotionally painful because when you despair, you cease your efforts and you lose any chance of achieving your goals.

Despair results from the feeling that you have lost control of your performance. Despair can have physical causes, for example, you sustain an injury, become dehydrated, are nutritionally deficient, or are experiencing significant pain. It can be caused by equipment problems, such as leaky goggles, getting multiple flats, or a persistent gear malfunction. Despair can arise in response to race conditions, for example, cold or rough water, an unrelenting headwind, or severe heat. It can occur due to psychological changes, for example, a significant loss of confidence following a poor swim or bike, failure to meet your pace expectations, or discouragement from being passed by many competitors. In all cases of despair, you feel that you've lost the ability to successfully pursue your goals and will be unable to regain that ability.

> *You get to a point where you can make the decision either way. If you go on, then you win. If you stop, you lose.*
>
> —John Collins,
> founder of Ironman

Finding the resolve to overcome despair may be your greatest emotional challenge as a triathlete. Mastering despair is difficult because you feel that you're at the very end of your rope and have little faith that you can recover. As with other emotions, mastering despair is a choice you make. This choice is not easy because your despair arises from not believing that you have a choice. We have found, however, that even in the worst situations, there are changes you can make to relieve the despair. You won't necessarily resolve the situation completely, but you can make changes that will ease your despair and keep you going.

Overcoming despair starts with understanding its causes. Perhaps the most difficult part of taking this first step is being able to step back from it far enough to look at your situation objectively. If you can detach yourself from your despair briefly, you can usually identify its cause. Once you know what's causing your despair, make changes to resolve it. In some cases, the cause can be addressed directly, for example, if you're dehydrated or calorie depleted, take a few extra minutes at an aid station to take in more fuel. Not all causes of despair can be solved directly, for example, your disappointment in having to walk during the run and realizing that you won't achieve your time goal. In these cases, you may need to adjust your goals. Even if you walk and don't reach your time goal, you can still benefit from continuing your effort, doing your best, and learning from the experience. Just finishing means you overcame adversity, gained mastery over your emotions, and didn't give up.

When you despair, your mind sends a message to your body to do the same. You can counter these feelings by creating physical changes that resist the decline in intensity using the psych-up techniques we describe in Chapter 5, including intense breathing, high-energy self-talk and body language, and intensity keywords. These strategies will produce a physical state that counters the feelings of letdown that accompany despair and will also spark your motivation and confidence.

POST-RACE DEPRESSION

Most everyone who has ever committed considerable time and energy to training and competing in a triathlon knows the feelings. During training and the race, you're motivated, excited, and energized. As you cross the finish line, you're psyched, elated, and joyous at having accomplished your goal. Up to that point, triathlon is fun. Then, a day or two later, it may hit you. You might feel down, lethargic, even sad. After a week, that malaise may still be there. You might even start to worry. You ask yourself, "Why am I so down?" You can try to resist it by getting back to your training, but this might just make it worse. You wonder if it will ever go away. You have been struck by "post-race depression" (PRD).

PRD is a common affliction that most triathletes (and, in fact, most endurance athletes) experience after big races. Such post-big-race down periods are natural and, despite triathletes' best efforts, usually unavoidable. The fact is, if you experience PRD, you shouldn't try to avoid these feelings. PRD plays an essential role in your continued physical and mental health. Yet PRD can be a source of uncertainty, concern, and just plain discomfort.

Any race that means something to you requires tremendous physical, psychological, and emotional investment. That investment causes you to put considerable time, energy, and effort into your training and to make substantial sacrifices in other parts of your life. In other words, your life becomes all about preparation for the big race. This investment, and the conclusion of your efforts, can lead to PRD. These down feelings are especially likely if you fail to achieve your competitive goals. This lack of "payoff" can create feelings of anger, frustration, and disappointment that can exacerbate the normal and healthy PRD that you would otherwise experience and can make recovery from PRD longer and more difficult.

When the big race is over, PRD may occur for several reasons. First, your body has been performing at a high level in training and then in the race for so long, it needs to take a break. Because it no longer needs to be up, your body shuts down. In fact, most of the "depression" (we don't mean it in the "I need to be on antidepressant medication" sense, which is extremely rare) is physiologically based. The body, in a sense, decides to take a brief vacation so it can rest and rejuvenate. As our thoughts and emotions are fundamentally physiological, this physical downturn also expresses itself mentally in "down" thoughts and emotions.

This so-called depression also has a direct psychological and emotional component. For months of training and during the competition, your goals, thoughts, and focus have had a clearly defined objective and direction; your life had purpose. With the event concluded, that purpose is gone and, along with it, is a short-term loss of a significant part of your self-identity (the part that is a triathlete). This lack of direction causes you to feel lost and rudderless. Questions such as "Who am I?" and "What now?" are common. You may question your recent performance, feel unmotivated, and be uncertain about your future as a triathlete.

An emotional letdown can be a powerful and uncomfortable part of PRD. After being on an emotional high—excitement, elation, joy—from the intense training and the race itself, the combination of the physiological decline and psychological loss of purpose often leads to down emotions, such as sadness, listlessness, irritability, and a general malaise. These emotions can be mild or quite severe depending on your personality, your experience with endurance sports, your coping skills, and how you performed in the recent race. It's not uncommon for triathletes with PRD to lose interest in other aspects of their lives, withdraw from previously enjoyable activities, feel sorry for themselves, and generally to do a lot of moping around, especially if they performed below expectations.

Given that some level of PRD is inevitable after big races, the key question is not how to avoid it, but rather how to deal with this uncomfortable post-event experience so that you can get through it as quickly as possible and use it to help you prepare for your next big race.

The first step in working through PRD is to accept that it is a normal and necessary part of triathlon. Allowing PRD to run its course and using it to your benefit will help you minimize both its severity and duration. PRD, though clearly uncomfortable, plays a vital role in your recovery from big races, much like a rest day after an intense week of training is essential to increased fitness. A common feeling with triathletes suffering from PRD is that it will never go away. This perception alone may cause you to feel even more down and make PRD worse. A part of the acceptance process is acknowledging that the feelings are okay and that they will pass in time.

As an active, goal-directed person, you may attempt to resist PRD by setting a new goal and returning to intense training before you're physically or psychologically ready. If you try this strategy, you may prolong the PRD. You're more likely to get sick, because your immune system functioning is down, or you may get injured because neither your body nor your mind are prepared for the renewed physical demands.

Instead, allow yourself to experience and naturally pass through the PRD. Be good to yourself. Ensure that you get extra rest, eat healthily, have a regular massage, take yoga, and try not to tax yourself too much. Enjoy not having a goal or direction. Revel in doing things you couldn't do when you were training—having weekends free, going to sleep after 9:00 P.M., drinking normal liquids instead of that awful energy drink, or eating a big, fat, juicy burger, curly fries, and an Oreo shake (okay, that's not healthy eating, but it tastes so good and you've earned it!)—and not doing all the things that you may have started to hate before your race—getting up for those early-morning masters swims, having your life revolve around your training. This "indulgence" will give your body the rest it craves and your spirit the lift it needs. It allows your mind and body to rejuvenate more quickly and enables you to return to your usual high-energy self sooner.

A difficult part of PRD is feeling like you've lost a part of yourself and, without training, you may feel "starved" for affirmation. Because you may not be "feeding" your physical self, turn your attention to other significant parts of yourself that you find nourishing, perhaps social or creative activities. This alternative "nutrition" will provide you with other meaningful sources of validation that will help you generate positive emotions to counteract your malaise and enable you to continue to feel good about yourself despite the absence of reinforcement from triathlon.

Lastly, do things that you enjoy simply for the experience—no goals, no purpose—for example, reading, going to movies, traveling. This experience is an essential part of keeping triathlon in perspective, gaining the most joy out of your participation and ensuring that you maintain some balance in your life despite your investment in triathlon. It also makes certain that, when you do return to training, you continue to participate for positive, healthy, and life-enriching reasons, and you're physically, psychologically, and emotionally ready to meet the challenges of the new goals you have set for yourself.

FOSTERING POSITIVE EMOTIONS

While the majority of this chapter has focused on negative emotions and how you can overcome them, learning to experience and express positive emotions is equally important. While negative emotions warn you when a problem may be arising, positive emotions show you what to seek out and look forward to. Enthusiasm, inspiration, pride, satisfaction, and happiness are the emotional goals toward which you should strive and are the emotional rewards for your efforts.

Experiencing and learning from positive emotions can also help you gain emotional mastery. You have opportunities on a daily basis to create, express, and share the positive emotions that you feel, particularly in training and races. There are no rules or techniques for benefiting from positive emotions. You will learn about positive emotions by allowing yourself to experience and express them. When you're excited about having had a great ride, focus on your excitement and let it engulf you. When you're inspired by someone else's efforts, tell them and allow yourself to feel the inspiration deeply. When you're thoroughly happy with your training or race, share it with someone and bask in its warmth. The more you acknowledge and experience your positive emotions, the more readily accessible they will be for you when you need them most.

TRIATHLETE SPOTLIGHT: GLORIA

Having been an avid biker and runner for many years, Gloria, age 38, was drawn to triathlon. There was just one minor problem: she was terrified of open-water swimming. Though she wasn't a bad swimmer technically and knew rationally that she wouldn't drown, just the thought of swimming in a lake—much less the ocean—was paralyzing to her. Cold, rough, murky water was her own personal idea of hell. At an open-water swim with her tri-club, Gloria had every intention of going in, but froze up before she got to the water. Her fear was palpable: heart racing, muscles tensed, shallow breathing, stomach stuck in her throat, eyes wide. Coaxing from other club members got her in up to her knees, but no farther. She sat and watched the other swimmers in the lake, relieved, but frustrated and ashamed.

Being a rather stubborn and prideful sort, Gloria was determined not to be beaten by her fear. She went to the Internet one evening and read everything she could about overcoming fear and put together a plan that she hoped would get her open-water swimming within four weeks. She had read that, with irrational fears, you could choose how you wanted to react, so she made a conscious and committed decision to face her fear and no longer allow it to intimidate her. She noticed that just making this strong statement gave her courage and resolve.

The first thing she did was post a question on her tri-club's Internet discussion group asking if any of its members were afraid of the water. To her surprise, most everyone said they had some fear of open-water swimming. Some of the club members offered her tips that helped them, which she noted and filed away for future use.

The coach in her masters program also said that fear of open water is commonplace. He said it usually comes from a lack of experience and confidence in one's swimming skills. The swim coach told her that she was a very competent swimmer and stated with absolute certainty that she was incapable of drowning in open water. The coach's faith in her gave her own confidence a little boost.

Gloria also learned that the physical symptoms of her fear were the most difficult to overcome because they were so powerful and immediate. She began to practice breathing and relaxation exercises before her masters swims to train her body to be more relaxed. She also regularly imagined herself entering and swimming in open water. At first, just imagining herself in open water was scary for her, but with each imagery

(continued on next page)

(continued from previous page)

session, she became increasingly comfortable with seeing and feeling herself swim. She also went to the lake every other day and just walked along its beach, getting her feet wet, and, as she put it, making friends with the open water.

After three weeks, Gloria decided she was ready for her first open-water swim. She chose to do it with just a few friends there to support her. She slowly waded in, stopping every few seconds to take some deep breaths and to relax her body. Though still scared, the feeling wasn't paralyzing. When she was in up to her waist, she turned parallel to the beach, took a deep breath, and started Tarzan swimming. At first she was stiff and uncomfortable, but within a few strokes, she started to loosen up. By focusing intently on her swim technique, she wasn't as aware of her fear. After about 50 yards, she stopped and stood up to the cheers from her friends. She then swam back to them, this time submerging her head and breathing from the side. She repeated this exercise several more times until she actually started to feel comfortable.

Gloria returned each day that week, gaining more confidence and comfort, and moving farther out from the shore. Each swim, she used the mental tools that she had learned, positive self-talk, relaxation exercises, and focusing techniques, to help her overcome the twinges of fear she still felt. On the last day of the fourth week since she began her quest, she led her tri-club teammates into the water, and she had never felt so proud.

CHAPTER

8 Pain

P ain is undoubtedly the greatest obstacle you face as a triathlete. Yet pain is also an essential and valuable part of triathlon training and competition. Pain lies at the top of the Prime Triathlon pyramid because it can be the ultimate determinant of whether you achieve your triathlon goals. Pain offers a powerful and persistent physical warning to your body that is difficult to ignore. Yet it also provides you with valuable information about your triathlon efforts that you can use to enhance your training and race experiences. Whether you use pain as an ally to pursue your triathlon goals or as an enemy to keep you from realizing your dreams depends on your understanding of pain and whether you can gain mastery over it.

PUTTING PAIN IN PERSPECTIVE

Using pain to your advantage starts with gaining a realistic perspective on the pain you experience as a triathlete. A few years ago, Jim was out for a long, hard ride with some friends. At the end of the ride, one of the guys said, "That was a sufferfest!" This declaration got Jim thinking about the pain triathletes feel and prompted him to explore the meaning of pain further and put it in a context that would help triathletes view pain realistically and deal with it effectively. This perspective starts with understanding the differences among suffering, pain, and physical discomfort.

Our work with the Leukemia and Lymphoma Society Team-in-Training groups has put training and competitive pain in perspective for us. What you experience in your triathlon training and racing is not suffering. People with cancer suffer because their pain is severe, long lasting, life threatening, and largely uncontrollable. What you feel in training and races may not even be true pain. True pain comes from injuries. This pain is similar to suffering, but injury pain—though sometimes severe—is not life threatening, typically doesn't last that long, and can be controlled much more easily.

You feel physical discomfort in training and races. It does hurt and it also interferes with your training and competitive efforts. But what you feel is entirely within your control—you can ease the discomfort anytime you want by simply slowing down or stopping. For simplicity's sake, though, you can continue to call what you experience pain because it is commonly used, but you'll now know what it really is, and that perspective is your first step to mastering pain.

> The swimming part—pretty much pain. The cycling part, well, you might catch a breath there. The running part is thirty minutes of constant pain. For the most part, the sport is about pain.
>
> —Hunter Kemper

Distinguishing Pain

For you to master the pain you experience in training and races, you need to distinguish between performance pain and injury pain. Performance pain is usually dull, more generalized, doesn't last long after exertion, produced voluntarily, entirely under your control, and can be reduced at will. Injury pain is typically severe or chronic, localized to a specific area, persisting after the conclusion of exertion, signaling danger to your health, and perceived as being outside of your control. These two diverse experiences of pain can produce markedly different physical, psychological, and emotional responses. Performance pain is often a source of satisfaction and inspiration, creating positive thoughts and emotions that can facilitate performance. Injury pain, on the other hand, can cause negative reactions, including loss of confidence and motivation, increased anxiety, and feelings of frustration and dread.

Providing you with these simple distinctions in the types of pain you experience in your triathlon efforts can help you to more clearly identify what kind of pain you're feeling in training and races. Your understanding of these differences can affect how you perceive (positively or negatively), evaluate (benign or harmful), and respond to (continued effort or ease up) your pain.

Interpreting Pain

The next step in overcoming triathlon pain is to understand that pain has two components that influence your experience of it. There is the physical experience of pain that you have to tolerate in your training and races. The pain you feel is real and communicates important information about your body. But you don't feel pain directly from your body. Pain has a major psychological component; your mind acts as a filter for the pain.

How you interpret pain, what you think about it, and the emotions you connect to it affect the pain you feel. How you interpret your pain can propel you to new and inspiring heights of performance or it can drag you to new lows of disappointment and despair.

▼

The most important thing I realized was, "You're not going to die—so just get on with it and deal with it."
—Dave Scott

Ignoring Pain

Some triathletes try to ignore the pain, their rationale being that if they don't think about it, then it won't affect them as much. So triathletes listen to music, talk to people they're training or racing with, or just think about other things. This form of distraction can work when pain first appears. This pain is not that severe yet and hasn't been around that long, so taking your mind off it can work initially. But ignoring pain as a long-term strategy is both ineffective and harmful. As pain grows and becomes more persistent, it's simply not possible to ignore it. The pain will insinuate itself into your mind and scream for it to be heard. Also, by ignoring pain, you're also ignoring what could be important information that you need to know about how your body is doing; for example, you may be going at an unsustainable pace or you've incurred an injury. There are times when it's okay to space out, such as on recovery rides or runs, but when you're putting in quality effort, for example, during speed work or in races, you want to be constantly monitoring your body and responding to what it's telling you.

Pain as Your Enemy

Pain becomes your enemy when you perceive it negatively, as something that is threatening to you and to be avoided. Negative thinking, such as "Pain is terrible," "Pain means I'm weak," and "Pain means I will fail," are common examples of negative perceptions of pain. Thinking of pain in this light may cause you to lose confidence and motivation, experience anxiety, and become consumed by the pain. When you're doing those 10 x 100s in the pool, hill repeats on your bike, or that 30-minute tempo run and you start thinking, "This hurts too much. I hate this. What am I doing out here?" this negative self-talk will actually increase the pain you feel, lessen your desire to fight through the pain, and limit the benefits you gain from training.

Some fascinating research has emerged recently that has found that the emotions that you connect with your pain have a significant impact on how much pain you feel. Like all triathletes, you've had the experience in a race when you're hurting. You begin to get frustrated that you won't reach your goal time. You get angry at yourself for not training harder. You may even despair of your ability to finish. When you connect these negative emotions with your pain in training or a race, you feel more pain.

Pain as Your Ally

Making pain your ally starts with recognizing that pain is a normal and necessary part of training and racing. Accept that it's going to hurt, a lot and for extended periods at times, rather than trying to avoid or fight it. If you're in pain, it means you're working hard and aggressively pursuing your goals. The more pain on the way to your goals, the more satisfaction you'll feel. In fact, if it didn't hurt, you probably wouldn't do triathlons. Also, realize that you're not the only one hurting out there. Everyone else is probably in as much pain as you are. There's a saying, "Misery loves company." This is not entirely true. The accurate adage is that, "Misery loves misery's company," meaning that we prefer to suffer when others around us are also suffering. So next time you're hurting in a race, look over at several of your competitors and realize that they're in a bad way too.

> *It takes a lot of mental prep for me to get ready to go to that level [of pain]. But it's knowing that the pain will end that keeps me going and knowing I will be happier at the finish if I do my absolute best that I can do on a given day.*
>
> —Pete Kain

Experience. Pain becomes your ally with experience. As a tri-newbie, the increasing amounts of pain you feel in your training and races may alarm you because these uncomfortable sensations are new to you. But the more miles you put in, the more you become familiar with it and the better you are able to adapt to and tolerate it. You learn how pain affects you physically and mentally. What does your body feel when you're in pain? How does your mind react to the pain? You also learn how to manage it—what reduces the pain, what makes it worse.

Pain as information. Staying emotionally detached from your pain can reduce the pain you feel. One way to disconnect from pain is to use your pain as information during training and races. Pain can offer you a wealth of valuable information that you can use to get the most out of your efforts. Pain tells you how hard you're working and whether what you're feeling is due to exertion or injury. Pain gives you direct information about your pace, technique, body position, posture, nutrition and hydration, and tactics. Responding to this information by, for example, adjusting your turnover during the swim, shifting from your aero bars to your drop bars or bullhorns every few miles, and altering your stride periodically will help you reduce your pain and maximize your performance.

I try to be aware of what is going on during my training and racing with my body. When I encounter discomfort, I try and figure out why it is happening and then what I can do to alleviate it. I think that it is most important to address the issue and then develop a plan that will hopefully fix the situation.

—Heather Fuhr

Relaxation. You can also take physical steps to reduce your pain. When your body begins to struggle, it tries to protect itself from the pain by tensing. Your body doesn't realize that this only makes it worse, so you need to tell it to relax. To combat the physical tension that comes with increasing pain, you can use the psych-down techniques we described in Chapter 5, such as deep breathing, relaxing your muscles, raising and lowering your shoulders, swinging your arms, shaking out your hands, keeping your face relaxed, and smiling. These simple strategies will help you induce a state of physical relaxation and can make a significant difference in how your body responds to pain.

Positive self-talk. Just as negative thoughts can cause you to feel more pain, positive self-talk can lessen the pain you feel. What you say to yourself about the pain you feel influences its intensity. Positive self-talk, such as "I'm getting stronger with every step," "This is making me tougher," and "I'm working toward my goals," not only reduces your pain, but it has other psychological benefits, including increased motivation, greater confidence, better focus, and more positive emotions.

Positive emotions. Connecting positive emotions, such as excitement and fulfillment, with the pain you feel in training and races reduces the pain and makes it more tolerable. Positive emotions create more positive self-talk and have other psychological advantages, such as greater motivation and confidence. Physiologically, positive emotions release endorphins (neurochemicals that act as internal painkillers) that not only reduce the perception of pain, but actually lessen the physical pain.

Given that you're in pain and not predisposed to feeling happy, what positive emotions can you generate that are realistic to the situation? We've found two that are powerful. Inspiration is our favorite positive emotion to experience when training and racing. You can view the pain you feel as part of an epic challenge to achieve your goals. Your pain tells you that you're working intensely and making progress toward your triathlon dreams. The more pain you feel, the more meaning, satisfaction, and joy you'll feel after your workout or race. To that end, we suggest a two-pronged strategy that combines generating positive self-talk and positive emotions. When you're in a lot of pain, for example, during a tough set of swim intervals or a long bike climb, smile and say, "Money in the bank, baby, money in the bank" (you have to say "baby" or it won't work). Reminding yourself of the reasons for your efforts will also cause you to feel inspired by the pain. The positive self-talk tells you that you're making deposits on your fitness that you'll be able to withdraw in races (unlike checking accounts, triathlons don't have overdraft protection). And smiling creates more positive emotions and releases those painkilling endorphins.

Pride is another emotion that you can realistically conjure up when you're in pain. Pride is the feeling of satisfaction in your efforts and

> *I usually tell myself that the pain will only last a bit longer, to just push a little more, for a little longer. I can usually outlast many of my competitors by doing this. I am usually ready to crack, but know if I can last for 10 more seconds, 20 more, and so on, that whomever I am next to may crack first.*
>
> —Pete Kain

accomplishments. When you're struggling during a workout or a race, focus on your ultimate goal, remember that the pain you're in is taking you another step toward it, and remind yourself how good you'll feel when you achieve that goal.

A quiet place. An experience that several pro triathletes, including Mark Allen, said they had involved going to a quiet place when they were really suffering. They described it as akin to an out-of-body experience in which they become an observer of their pain rather than experiencing it directly. This mental and emotional disconnection from their pain usually occurred late in races when they were at the limits of their ability to withstand the pain. All of the triathletes noted that this shift in their experience of the pain occurred naturally rather than by design. One minute, their body was in agony from their effort and their mind was screaming for it to stop. Another minute they experienced a shift in which the pain, though still present, seemed to be at a distance—felt, but only indirectly—and the noise in their mind ceased. This quiet place allowed them to maintain their effort and finish strong.

You know it's going to be over in a few minutes, and my mind would cross over while my body took over. Everything went quiet. The pain was so intense that I moved beyond it and my mind just shut off. Pain isn't pain anymore. I came to this place with a lot of racing. Every time I came to that place of quiet, I knew I could survive, I could go back to it each race, as painful as it was.

—Mike Pigg

Essential lesson. Finally, perhaps the greatest lesson we've learned about the relationship between pain and triathlon performance is this: The physical pain you feel in training and races pales in comparison to the emotional pain you'll feel if you don't achieve your goals because you didn't master the pain. The pain you feel during the race is temporary, but the feelings of accomplishment and pride you feel at the finish line having overcome that pain will last forever.

TRIATHLETE SPOTLIGHT: MELISSA

Melissa, a 24-year-old who has been doing triathlons for two years, felt like she had a really low threshold for pain compared to the women she trained with. Even though she seemed to be in as good a shape as most of them, she was the one who always broke down first on long hills or during track workouts. Growing up, she was aware of how sensitive she was to pain, recalling the pain she felt at the dentist or when she had to get a shot at the doctor's office. In training and races, she would start to hurt and, though she would try to resist it, she always gave in to the pain and eased up.

A member of her local tri-club, Steve, was a psychologist, so she asked him if her inability to deal with her pain was mental or physical. He said that it may be both. People do seem to be wired with varying degrees of sensitivity to pain and that can't be changed. This news was discouraging to Melissa, but Steve went on to say that pain tolerance can be increased using a few simple techniques. As they both participated in the club's Tuesday evening track workouts, which are routinely painful, Steve suggested that they approach her pain in two steps.

At the next Tuesday night workout, Steve asked Melissa to monitor her physiology, thoughts, and emotions when she started to hurt during the evening's intervals. At the end of the session, they sat down and she described what she experienced. She noticed, first of all, that toward the end of an interval, her shoulders would tighten up and she would start to lose her form. She also became aware that when the pain first arose, she would start thinking really negatively. Finally, she told Steve that she would get really frustrated and mad at herself when it began to hurt a lot.

Between that evening and next Tuesday, Steve suggested several exercises. He wanted her to lie down each day and imagine herself giving her best effort while running an 800-meter interval and see and feel herself running comfortably and with manageable pain. On her longer runs during the week, he also asked her to replay a song in her head that made her feel good.

The next Tuesday workout involved 8 x 800-meter repeats. Steve asked Melissa to divide the workout into four sets of two intervals each. For the first two 800s, she should focus on her body, keeping her shoulders relaxed and down, breathing in a controlled way, and maintaining her form and stride, particularly during the last 200 meters when it got difficult. After the two intervals, Melissa told Steve that, even though her effort was the same as at last week's workout, she felt more relaxed and thought she was able to maintain her stride better.

On the second set of 800s, Steve wanted Melissa to focus on her thoughts, in particular, being aware when negative thoughts arose and immediately replacing them with positive self-talk. He asked her to think of two positive thoughts that she could use and she came up with, "I am strong" and "Finish fast." Following this set, Melissa said that the positive self-talk overrode the negative thoughts and she didn't feel like she was dragging a tire the last half lap like she had in the past.

For the third set of 800s, Steve asked Melissa to be aware of her emotions during the intervals and, when she started to feel frustration, to replace them with positive emotions. He suggested that when it started to hurt, she should smile and generate feelings of inspiration from giving her best effort as she pursued her goals. She ran up to Steve with a big smile on her face after the set and told him that she felt completely different on those intervals—light, fast, and happy.

On the final set of 800s, Steve had Melissa simply sing her song throughout each interval and see what thoughts, emotions, and physical effects occurred. After the two intervals, she told Steve that she had never run her 800s so fast before. Singing the song caused her to relax, think more positively, and create good emotions. The workout still hurt plenty, but the exercises Steve had her do took the edge off of the pain so it was something that she could deal with. She couldn't wait to try out her newfound pain tolerance in a race.

PART THREE

Tools for
Triathlon Success

CHAPTER

9 Goal Setting and Mental Training Plans

Motivation is not enough to become your best. Motivation without goals is like knowing where you want to go without knowing how to get there. Goals act as the road map to your desired destination. Goals increase your commitment and motivation, provide deliberate steps toward your triathlon aspirations, and allow you to track your progress.

A goal-setting program begins with a vision of what you want to accomplish in the sport. Your vision may be to make it through an Olympic-distance race, do a half-Ironman, finish an Ironman, or qualify for Kona. A vision provides a clear why, what, where, and how for your triathlon efforts. The Prime Triathlon Goal Formula (see below) illustrates the important role that goals perform in realizing your vision.

PRIME TRIATHLON GOAL FORMULA

VISION + MOTIVATION + GOALS = PROGRESS

TYPES OF GOALS

The effectiveness of a goal-setting program doesn't just depend on setting goals, but also on setting the correct types of goals that will take you from where you are now to where you want to be in the future. There are seven types of goals you should set in your goal-setting program:

1. *Long-term* goals represent what you ultimately want to achieve in triathlon, such as continue to show improvements in your fitness and your race times, to finish a certain distance race, stand on the podium at a local triathlon, qualify for an age-group championship, or race as a professional.

2. *Yearly* goals indicate what you want to achieve in the next twelve months, for example, to achieve a certain race time, attain a particular ranking, or qualify for a specific race.

3. *Race* goals specify how you want to perform in races you'll be competing in during the coming year.

> *I definitely don't see getting on the medal stand as something that's unattainable. I see it as a lofty goal. What I'm trying to focus on is going out and competing against my fellow competitors, the racecourse, and myself. I'm going to give my best effort, and if it warrants a podium finish, that's what it warrants.*
> —Andy Potts

4. *Feeling* goals represent how you want to feel in or about a race, for example, "I want to race comfortably," "I want to finish strong," and "I want to have a great time in the race."

5. *Training* goals identify what you need to do in your physical, technical, tactical, and mental training to achieve your competitive goals.

6. *Lifestyle* goals indicate what you need to do in your general lifestyle to reach your goals, such as sleep, diet, work or school, and relationships.

7. *Fulfillment* goals specify what you want to get out of your triathlon experiences, for example, improved health and fitness, enjoyment, challenge, friendships, or results.

The first three goals, long-term, yearly, and race, can be categorized as *outcome* goals because they describe specific results you want to achieve.

Outcome goals are important because they provide the destinations of your goal-setting program. Once you set your outcome goals, you should place them out in the distance as what you ultimately want to achieve. Remembering your outcome goals can help motivate you when your training gets difficult and you start to wonder whether your efforts are worth it. But some triathletes become so focused on their outcome goals that it actually interferes with achieving these goals. Becoming obsessed with achieving certain results can keep you from focusing on what you need to do to reach those outcome goals and take the fun out of your training and races.

The latter four goals, feeling, training, lifestyle, and fulfillment, are *process* goals and should be your primary focus in your day-to-day training efforts. By focusing on your process goals, you'll ensure that you do what needs to be done to reach your outcome goals. Your emphasis on the process of your triathlon preparations will make pursuing your outcome goals more manageable, enable you to focus on the enjoyment of triathlon, and ensure that you get the most quality out of your efforts.

I set certain goals each year for my training and racing. Some of these goals are quantitative—wanting to try and swim a certain time, do well at a specific race, and so on. Other goals are more qualitative in nature— wanting to get stronger in a certain discipline, build more strength in the gym, and so on. Goals, whether qualitative or quantitative, give us something to focus on—something that all the hard work, day in day out, is gearing toward. Without these goals, sometimes there seems to be a lack of direction in my training.

—Heather Fuhr

GOAL GUIDELINES

The effectiveness of your goal-setting program depends on whether you understand what kinds of goals to set and how to use them to enhance your motivation and direction. There are seven goal guidelines you should follow to get the most out of your goal setting.

1. **Process goals should build to outcome goals.**

   Process goals lead progressively to outcome goals. For example, your lifestyle goals (e.g., being rested and eating well) should help you accomplish your training goals (e.g., increase your speed and stamina), which, in turn, should lead to your race goals (e.g., race times and placings), which should enable you to reach your yearly goals (e.g., complete a new race distance or year-end ranking), which, finally, should allow you to achieve your long-term goals (e.g., complete an Ironman or qualify for nationals). Following this progression will ensure that your process goals always support and encourage achievement of your outcome goals.

2. **Goals should be challenging, but realistic and attainable.**
   Set goals that you can realistically attain, but only with time and effort. If you set goals that are too easy, you'll reach them with little effort, so they'll do little for your motivation and progress as a triathlete. If you set goals that are too difficult, you won't be able to achieve them, which can also discourage motivation and progress.

3. **Goals should be specific and concrete.**
   It's not sufficient to set a goal such as "I want to improve my running speed this year." Goals should be clearly stated and measurable. For example, "I want to increase my speed in my 800 repeats on the track by five seconds over three months." This goal indicates the precise area to be worked on, the specific amount of improvement aimed for, and the time frame in which to achieve the goal.

4. **Focus on degree of, rather than absolute, goal attainment.**
   An inevitable part of goal setting is that you won't reach all of your goals, because it's not possible to accurately judge what is realistic for all goals. Be concerned with how much of the goal you achieve (i.e., degree of attainment) rather than whether or not you fully reach the goal (i.e., absolute attainment). Though you won't attain all of your goals, you will almost always improve toward a goal. With this perspective, if you don't reach a goal, but still improve 50 percent over the previous level, you're more likely to view yourself as having been successful in achieving the goal.

5. **Goal setting is dynamic and fluid.**
   Goal setting is a process that never ends. When one goal is achieved, set another goal that is higher or in a different area to continually

encourage yourself to improve. Review your goals regularly, compare them to your actual progress, and adjust them as needed. Because you won't be able to set goals with perfect accuracy, be open to making changes as needed. For example, goals that you reach more easily than expected should be immediately reset to a higher level. Conversely, if you set goals that were too difficult to achieve, modify them to a more realistic level.

6. **Prepare a written contract.**
   Research suggests that goal setting is most effective when it's prepared as a written contract comprised of explicit statements of your goals and the specific ways you'll achieve them. This approach clearly identifies your goals and holds you accountable for the fulfillment of the contract. You can complete a goal-setting contract, sign it, and give copies to your coach, training buddies, family, or friends. To ensure that you continue to follow the contract, you should periodically review the contract and determine whether you're continuing to pursue the goals stated in the contract.

7. **Chart your progress.**
   The most motivating aspect of goal setting is working toward and achieving the goals you establish. There is immense satisfaction and validation in seeing that your efforts are being rewarded with improvement. To foster these positive feelings, chart your progress in different parts of your training. For example, record your times for your 100-yard swim intervals, track your resting heart rate, or chart the increases in your cycling distances.

You can gain regular feedback about how you're doing in pursuing your goals from a number of sources. Feedback about your progress can come from coaches, video analysis, physical testing, or with Prime Triathlon profiling (see Chapter 2). Consistent feedback showing your improvement in various aspects of your training bolsters your motivation by showing you that your efforts are resulting in progress toward your goals.

Using the Prime Triathlon Goal Setting form (see pages 126 and 127), write down your goals following the goal guidelines just described. If you're uncertain of what your goals should be, ask your coach, your trainer, or others who know what you're working toward.

PRIME TRIATHLON GOAL SETTING, PART 1

Directions: In the space below, indicate your long-term, yearly, race, and feeling goals.

Long-Term (ultimate triathlon goal):

Yearly (performance and ranking goals for the year):

Race (goals for specific races):

Feeling (goals about how you want to feel):

KEY RACE GOALS

When we ask triathletes what their goals are for a particular race, their responses usually relate to a particular result they want to achieve, such as a time or placing: "I want to finish in the top fifteen in my age group," "I want to beat my training partner," or "I want to finish in less than three hours." But before you set an outcome goal, there are several other goals you should aim for that will help you achieve that great finish you're looking for.

Race goal #1: Get to the start. Your first race goal should be to get through your training program and arrive at the race fit, rested, injury and

PRIME TRIATHLON GOAL SETTING, PART 2

Directions: In the space below, set your technical, physical, mental, and lifestyle goals that will enable you to achieve your race, yearly, and long-term goals. Also, under method, indicate specifically how you will reach your training and lifestyle goals.

TRAINING (GOALS FOR ALL ASPECTS OF PREPARATION):

Technical (biomechanics, tactics):

1.   Method:

2.   Method:

3.   Method:

Physical (endurance, strength, flexibility):

1.   Method:

2.   Method:

3.   Method:

Mental (motivation, confidence, intensity, focus, emotions):

1.   Method:

2.   Method:

3.   Method:

Lifestyle (sleep, diet, work/school, relationships):

1.   Method:

2.   Method:

3.   Method:

illness free, and having enjoyed your training experience. This goal may seem obvious, but we meet many triathletes who had to miss a race or arrived unprepared because they were overtrained, injured, sick, or so tired of the training that they weren't going to enjoy their race.

Race goal #2: Be totally prepared. Your next race goal is to come to the start line ready to race. Jim was fortunate enough to work with a number of endurance athletes who competed in the 2000 Olympic Games in Sydney. At their last pre-Olympic training camp, he told them that when they got to the start line, they wanted to be able to say to themselves, "I am as prepared as I can be for this race." You can't control everything that happens in a race, for example, weather and course conditions, other competitors' performances, or mechanical problems, but being as prepared as you can puts you in a position to perform your best. Making this statement means that you've put in the necessary time and effort in your physical, technical, tactical, and mental training to achieve your race goals.

Race goal #3: Race Smart. This goal involves racing a smart tactical race. It means sticking with your race plan, staying on pace or within your heart rate ranges, and not getting pulled into a change in tactics because of how you feel at the moment or what other competitors are doing. Your goal is to swim, bike, and run at a pace you trained for and that allows you to maintain that pace consistently start to finish.

For your A-priority races, include three different goals: (1) a great day, which may include variable weather conditions, broken goggles, a flat tire, and digestive problems; (2) a fantastic day, in which only half of those problems occur; and (3) a brilliant day, where the race goes as planned in your best scenario.... This will allow a little psychological latitude in dealing with a solid, but not necessarily perfect result.

—Dave Scott

Race goal #4: Finish strong. You also want a race goal for the end of the race. Your goal should be to have enough energy at the end of the race to be able to pick up the pace, pass people, and to finish strong. There is nothing more inspiring and exciting than having enough fuel in your tank to put on a kick and use the energy of the racers you're passing to propel you to the finish.

Race goal #5: Enjoy the race. One goal that most triathletes don't even think about, but that we recommend strongly is: "Revel in the experience!" During the race, the most important goal you should strive for is to gain immense satisfaction and enjoyment out of the experience. Even when it's difficult, when you're tired and hurting, remember why you do it and enjoy the race.

Race goal #6: See results. Only then, after accomplishing all of your other race goals, focus on your outcome goal for the race. Remember that your result occurs at the end of the race, so focusing on it during the race will only distract you from your other goals. When you cross the finish line and have taken a moment to revel in finishing, only then can you look at the clock and see whether you achieved your outcome goal.

MENTAL TRAINING PROGRAM

You now know what your goals are and what you need to work toward. The aim of the mental training program is to help you achieve these goals in the most efficient and organized way possible. You can develop your own individualized mental training program by following three steps: design, implementation, and maintenance.

Design

The first thing to do in the *design* phase of developing your mental training program is to identify your

There's no question, the component of triathlon training that is lagging behind is the mental component. We haven't done a very good job of integrating psychology into training programs.

—Dave Scott

most crucial needs. Use the results from your Prime Triathlon profile (from Chapter 2), as well as physical testing, coaches' feedback, and your own training and race experience, to help you specify the areas in which you need the most work. You'll also have different areas you need to work on in the different triathlon disciplines. For example, staying focused in the water may be most important in your swimming, staying relaxed may be most necessary on the bike, and mastering pain may be most critical in your running. Using the Prime Triathlon Identification form on page 131, list the areas in which to focus in various aspects of your training and racing.

The next thing to do in designing your mental training program is to specify particular training strategies used to develop the areas you've just identified. For example, if you've set goals to improve your confidence, we described six strategies in Chapter 4 you could use. Narrow those choices to two or three techniques that you like most. To do this, experiment with the different techniques for a few days and see which ones you're most comfortable with. You can use the same approach with your physical

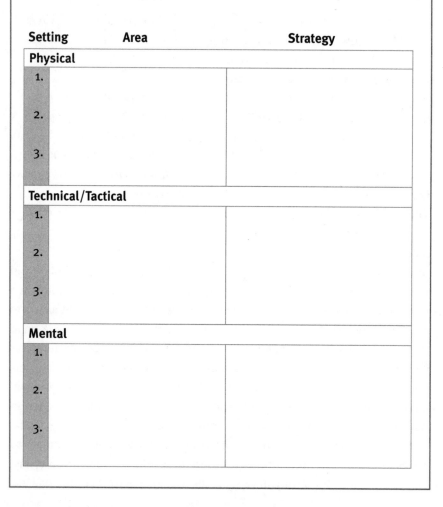

PRIME TRIATHLON IDENTIFICATION FORM

Directions: In the space below, indicate the training areas on which you need to work in the different settings. Then, specify strategies you will use to develop these areas.

Setting	Area	Strategy
Physical		
1.		
2.		
3.		
Technical/Tactical		
1.		
2.		
3.		
Mental		
1.		
2.		
3.		

technical training. Once again using the Prime Triathlon Identification form, list the two or three techniques you've chosen.

The final part of the design phase is to organize your mental training program into a daily and weekly schedule. This step should incorporate your physical, technical, and mental training into an organized plan. The Sample Prime Triathlon Mental Training Program below illustrates how you can organize mental training techniques into a cohesive program. Using the Prime Triathlon Planner on page 133, lay out the training program that addresses key aspects of the preparations you've specified in the Prime Triathlon Identification form.

TABLE **9.1** SAMPLE PRIME TRIATHLON MENTAL TRAINING PROGRAM

GOAL	STRATEGY	PLACE IN SCHEDULE
Increase motivation	Goal setting	Every Monday
Build confidence	Positive self-talk	In training and races
Increase focus	Keywords	Tuesday track
Master pain	Deep breathing, muscle relaxation	During rides and runs

Implementation

The second phase of the mental training program is *implementation*. This is where you put into action the plan you've just designed. It's best that you begin the program as far in advance of triathlon season as possible. There are several benefits to starting your program early. It enables you to develop the most effective mental training program possible and incorporate it fully into your overall training program. It lets you fine-tune the program to best suit your needs. Most importantly, it gives you the time to improve and gain its benefits.

A concern you may have is the time commitment required for a mental training program. Even without triathlon, you probably lead a busy life filled with work, family, and friends. Adding a comprehensive mental training program to your busy life may seem overwhelming. As you establish

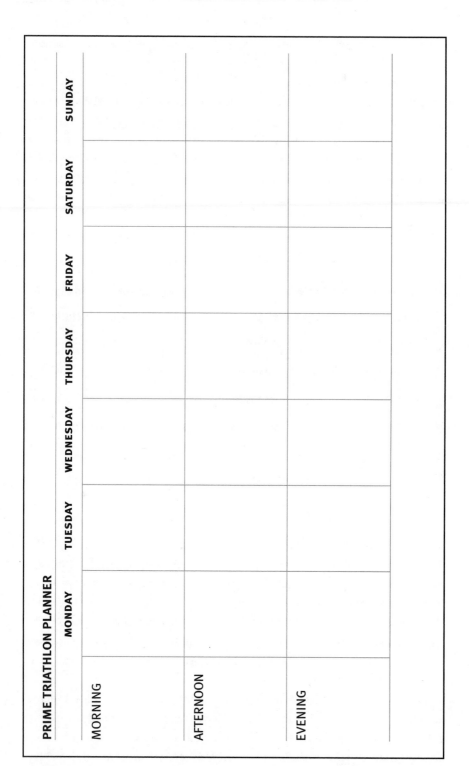

PRIME TRIATHLON PLANNER

	MONDAY	TUESDAY	WEDNESDAY	THURSDAY	FRIDAY	SATURDAY	SUNDAY
MORNING							
AFTERNOON							
EVENING							

goals and create a mental training program to meet those goals, consider what is realistic given the life you lead. If you feel that the program you've created is simply too much for you, it's better to start small rather than begin a time- and energy-consuming program that is impractical for you to manage. Reduce your program to its most essential elements, allowing you to improve and progress toward your goals. As you settle into the program and schedule it into your overall life, you can see whether it is manageable. If you find that your mental training program fits into your life, consider adding elements that will accelerate your progress or that will address other areas in need of improvement.

Maintenance

The final phase of the mental training program is *maintenance*. In triathlon, training doesn't ever have to stop. To continue to improve, you must maintain a consistent training program that addresses all aspects of the sport. Physical conditioning and technical skills will atrophy if they're not maintained through regular use. The same holds true for mental skills. Once you've developed the mental skills that will allow you to achieve your triathlon goals for the season, you can adjust your mental training program to ensure maintenance of that level.

Your commitment to triathlon and your desire to raise your goals at the start of each new season will determine the intensity of your mental training program during the off-season. Some triathletes don't do mental training during the entire off-season, requiring them to regain their previous season's mental skills each year. Others maintain a moderate level of mental training that provides them with a consistent base from which they can build when the new season starts. Still others use the off-season to gain mental strength and alleviate weaknesses, so they continue a rigorous mental training program that takes them to a new level of "mental fitness" for the new triathlon season.

TRIATHLETE SPOTLIGHT: RAY

Ray, a 44-year-old, had been progressing steadily since he took up the sport three years ago, despite the fact that he had no real goals each season. He just did races because they were fun and mostly just liked hanging out with healthy people. He started to wonder how fast he could go if he became "a man with a plan" and decided to set some real goals toward which he could work. Using an article on goal setting he had read recently, he laid out his goal-setting program.

Ray first decided that his long-term goal would be to complete an Ironman, though he felt like that objective was several years away. His yearly goal was to be fit enough to be able to finish his first half-Ironman in early September. He had several race goals, including an early-season warm-up sprint and three Olympic-distance races to prepare him for the half-Ironman. His feeling goal was to feel relaxed and comfortable during races and not suffer too much late in races. His training goals over the next three months included improving his 100s in the pool by ten seconds, increasing his bike mileage by 40 miles, and running fifteen seconds faster in his 800-meter track intervals. Ray's lifestyle goals included cutting out dessert four days a week, going to bed by 11:00 P.M. every weeknight, and not working on weekends. Finally, his fulfillment goals included succeeding at these new challenges and enjoying himself even though he was taking triathlon more seriously than before.

Being a self-described "head case," Ray was really into organizing a mental training program to help him through his triathlon season. The three mental areas he wanted to work on were focus and intensity in training and dealing with pain. Because he found swimming kind of boring and his workouts often lost their focus and intensity after a short time, he chose to improve those two areas during his masters swims. Every time he got into the pool, he had a keyword to focus on that would help his swimming and keep him from drifting away. He also used psych-up self-talk to keep his intensity high while swimming.

Ray suffered the most on the bike, so he decided that he would practice his pain-management techniques during his Wednesday hill repeats and his long Saturday rides. For the repeats, he used positive self-talk, deep breathing, and feelings of inspiration when he started to hurt. On the Saturday rides, he focused on staying relaxed, changing his body position on the bike, and shaking out his arms and hands periodically.

As the race season progressed, Ray was aware of how much his mental skills had improved. The quality of his swim training had gotten much better and his 100-yard times reflected it. His pain threshold seemed to have gotten higher too. He was able to tolerate much more pain during his hill repeats, and his average speed in his long rides reflected this improvement. With his first half-Ironman approaching, he never felt better prepared to achieve his goals.

CHAPTER

10 Training

uccess in triathlon doesn't happen on the day of the race, just before the race, or even during the race. Success comes from the days, weeks, and months of training that prepare you for the race. What you do in training will determine how you perform and the ultimate outcome of the event. Training is where the development of Prime Triathlon begins. It's the place where all of the physical, technical, tactical, and mental requirements of triathlon are established. Your goal in your training efforts is to achieve prime training, which we define as maintaining consistently high-quality training, resulting in optimal preparation to achieve your triathlon goals. Prime training comes from applying the highest level of effort, focus, and intensity throughout your workouts.

POSITIVE CHANGE FORMULA

Change of any sort, whether physical, technical, tactical, or mental, doesn't occur automatically. There is a three-step process, what we call the Positive Change Formula, that will enable you to be optimally prepared to achieve your triathlon goals in the quickest and most efficient way possible. First, become aware of what you need to work on and how to improve it. This awareness comes from physical testing, video analysis, feedback from coaches or training partners, and a general understanding of what you need to do to achieve your goals. Second, put in the time that will allow you to gain the necessary fitness and skills. There is no shortcut to progress in triathlon. You have to put in the time and energy swimming, biking, and running to see improvement. Finally, ensure that you instill quality into your training, which means having a clear purpose in your workouts and applying the necessary focus and intensity to maximize the benefits you gain from your efforts. Developing your triathlon capabilities involves an awareness of your physical, technical, tactical, and mental capabilities, and putting in sufficient quality time in the pool, on your bike, running, and in the weight room to gain the fitness and skills you need.

POSITIVE CHANGE FORMULA

AWARENESS + TIME + QUALITY = POSITIVE CHANGE

PRIME TRAINING

For you to get the most out of your training, have a clear idea of what you're doing at every workout and what you want to accomplish, for example, going onto the track knowing how many intervals you're going to run and at what pace. With this understanding you'll put in the time and have the quality you need to maximize the value of your training time and gain the benefits from your efforts. To get the most out of your training, adhere to the following guidelines.

Training has reached a new level for me right now; I have high expectations when I go into a workout. Old performances are no longer acceptable.

—Andy Potts

Goal and Purpose

Train with a goal and a purpose. A goal is some aspect of triathlon that you want to improve, such as a physical, technical, tactical, or mental area. A purpose is something specific you work on in training that will enable you to achieve your goal. For example, if your goal is to improve your power on the bike, your purpose might be to do six sets of one-mile climbs at 150 heartbeats per minute. Or if your goal is to improve your swimming efficiency, your purpose might be to do 500 yards of drills every swim workout.

100-percent Focus and Intensity

Another area in which most triathletes need work is their focus and intensity in training. Train at a level of focus and intensity that will allow you to perform your best in races. The focus and intensity that you bring to a race depends on your focus and intensity in training. Ideally, you want to train at 100-percent focus and intensity. When we talk about 100-percent focus and intensity, we don't mean going all out at your anaerobic threshold every workout. We mean that, whatever your goal and purpose for the workout, you should be totally focused on accomplishing that goal and purpose with no distractions or lapses, and you should put all of your effort and energy into that goal and purpose. For example, if your goal is to become more efficient on your bike and your purpose is to ride 50 miles keeping your heart rate at your aerobic threshold, then you should be entirely focused on maintaining that pace and your effort should be directed at staying there consistently. When you have sufficient focus and intensity, you're guaranteeing yourself quality training time and the benefits that result. You also make it easier to reach 100-percent focus and intensity in races because your mind and body become accustomed to that level of focus and intensity from training.

The adversity makes it so fun. If there's a hurricane and we have 3-foot swells, I'd think, "Damn, I have to learn to swim through that kind of wave." I always saw such conditions as a great opportunity, always loved headwinds and tailwinds. In Kona you'd be doing 18 mph in a headwind, then you'd turn around and do 45. And I would always think, "How can I make this situation better, how can I squeeze another half mile per hour out of this?" Training a lot on my own really helped. You have to push through on your own; it made me tough. Training on steep hills or in rain or headwinds in Humboldt County [California] made me tough. There's so much conversation around the conditions before races, I would always think, "Just take care of yourself and deal with it, just deal with it."

—Mike Pigg

Train for Adversity

As we suggested in Chapter 4 with respect to confidence, an essential skill to develop is to respond positively to adversity. Most triathletes like to train in ideal conditions, for example, warm water, smooth, flat roads, and no wind, yet conditions are rarely perfect in races. Too often in training, we see triathletes put forth less effort or stop completely when the conditions get too difficult. You might say it doesn't matter because it's just training. But the attitudes and habits you develop in training will come out in races. If you let up or give up in training when things get too tough, then you're ingraining that habit in the face of adversity. That reaction will come out when you're faced with adversity in races.

The way to learn to react positively to adversity in races is to train in and respond positively to those challenging conditions. A positive reaction to adversity comes from accepting the conditions and realizing that everyone else in the race has to deal with the difficult conditions as well. A part of this positive reaction is not allowing yourself to become frustrated because your performance declines. Stay positive and motivated even when the conditions are challenging. By training for adversity, you also come to understand the adverse conditions and learn how to adapt yourself to them, for example, adjusting your pace in a headwind or drinking more on a hot day. Having trained for adversity, when you compete in adverse conditions, you can say, "I've been training in these conditions. I know how to handle them," and you can have a good race despite the conditions.

> *I recall at least a couple of Hawaii Ironmans® when I got to the edge of pushing and didn't think I could push through that place. I felt I could have run faster retrospectively. I do feel like I sometimes didn't push past that place into new territory— not sure I ever did that like some of the other guys were doing. It was too uncomfortable for me. Sometimes I didn't throw down like I should have.*
>
> —Paul Huddle

Get Out of Your Comfort Zone

Triathlon training is not always easy. In fact, it can be downright painful a good part of the time. But staying in your comfort zone will keep you from improving. To become your best, you must move out of your comfort zone, which means challenging yourself to go beyond the effort you usually give and the pain you feel in training. It involves seeking areas in need of improvement and spending extra time on them, even if it's boring or painful. It means putting yourself in situations that you would normally avoid, such as cold open-water swims, but that you must face to improve. The risk of moving out of your comfort zone is that it may feel bad, and you'll be focusing on things that you're not good at or in which you lack confidence. But as you spend more time outside of your comfort zone, a funny thing happens; your comfort zone gets bigger until you reach a point at which it's no longer uncomfortable. Before you know it, you've expanded your comfort zone and taken your performances to a new level.

Never Give Up

Because triathlon training is so demanding, there may be times when you want to give up. Perhaps you've been dropped by the group you're riding with or you're in pain after the sixth of ten 800-meter track intervals. You might shorten your workout, reduce your effort, or stop altogether. You might rationalize giving up by saying that training doesn't really count and that you'd never give up in a race. But training matters a great deal because everything you do in training either contributes to or interferes with you gaining the maximum benefit your training program allows. Also, when you give up repeatedly, you're training yourself to give up when things get tough and your learned reaction in a race may then be to give up.

The habit of never giving up is critical because something rather important happens every time you give up; you automatically fail. If you continue to try through the difficulties, you may not fully achieve your goals, but at least you will gain satisfaction from your ongoing efforts. Overcoming difficult conditions is a source of great pride and inspiration, and you'll be motivated to overcome other challenges in the future. When

Most of us have, at some point, considered dropping out of a race. It's never an easy decision to make, and it's often the right one, but unless you're risking your health by finishing, it's almost always better to tough it out—even if that means walking to the finish with a group of like-minded folks. Through personal experience, I've found that after you drop out once, it becomes a lot easier to do the next time. A few years ago, I did almost an entire season of dropping out of races. Finally, 1997 Ironman world champion Thomas Hellriegel came up to me after a race and said, "Never drop out, because if you finish, your legs hurt for a week, but if you drop out, your head hurts for a month."

—Peter Reid

you resist the urge to give up when things get tough, you've won an even more important battle, namely, the one against yourself.

EIGHT LAWS OF PRIME PREPARATION

As we discussed in Chapter 3, motivation pushes you to put in the necessary time and effort to be your best. This time and effort ensures that you have prime preparation, which we define as doing everything you can to be fully prepared to perform your best. Preparation acts as the bridge between prime motivation and Prime Triathlon. Without preparation, you won't have the fitness, skills, or experience to achieve your triathlon goals. From our years of working with triathletes at all levels of ability, as well as our own endurance sport experience, we've developed eight laws that you must understand and follow to accomplish prime preparation and achieve Prime Triathlon.

First Law: Take responsibility for everything that can influence your triathlon performance. Prime preparation can be achieved if you know every area that affects your triathlon performance, including all of the components of physical, technical, tactical, and mental preparation. If you address every one of these areas, you can be sure that when you get to a race, you will be totally prepared to perform your best.

Second Law: Prime Triathlon is about "the grind." To be your best, you have to commit a great deal of time to your training. We call this the grind, which involves having to put hours upon hours into training, well beyond the point that it is fun and exciting. The grind can be boring, tiring, and painful. But if you accept the grind and focus on the positive aspects of your training, such as the satisfaction in your efforts and progress toward your goals, your motivation will sustain itself.

Third Law: Prime Triathlon requires that you train smart. Triathlon places incredible physical demands on you. Training requires that you put in large amounts of mileage swimming, biking, and running. The ability to strike the balance between not training enough and training too much is what will determine whether you achieve your triathlon goals. Some triathletes believe that simply putting in the miles will be enough. But junk miles lack quality and the benefits will be limited. Other triathletes believe that more is better. If you buy into this attitude, you may overtrain, burn out, or become injured. Training smart involves having a well-thought-out training program that emphasizes both quantity and quality, and has an effective mix of volume, intensity, and recovery, and listening to your body.

Fourth Law: The purpose of training is to develop effective competitive skills and habits. Triathlon training is much more than gaining cardiovascular fitness and sound swimming, biking, and running technique. Training must instill in you the competitive skills and habits that will enable you to fully use the physical fitness and technical skills you've ingrained. Essential competitive skills and habits encompass many of the issues we discuss in this book, including motivation and confidence in the face of adversity, staying relaxed and focused throughout a race, maintaining control of your emotions late in races, and being able to master the pain you will inevitably feel as you push yourself to achieve your goals.

Put yourself in critical situations in training to learn to be calm in critical situations in races. They force you to focus and get the job done. Once you've been through things that are stressful and unfamiliar, it's not a big deal in races. This allows me to be calm and work the problems in a race and maintain my composure.

—Victor Plata

Fifth Law: Consistent training leads to consistent race performance. Consistency is a hallmark of Prime Triathlon and is one of the most important qualities that put the best triathletes above the rest. Consistency in a race comes from consistency in training. Consistency relates to every aspect of triathlon training and life. In addition to the obvious areas, such as conditioning, technique, and tactics, it also pertains to attitude, effort, focus, intensity, emotions, sleep, diet, and lifestyle. Any area that influences your performance must be consistent before you can expect to perform consistently in a race.

Sixth Law: Patience and persistence are essential for Prime Triathlon. Triathlon fitness takes time to develop. You may become impatient and try to "fast forward" your training by working longer and harder. You'll experience plateaus and down periods along the way. You may become frustrated with these setbacks and want to quit. If you let impatience and frustration overwhelm you, you will never achieve Prime Triathlon. If you understand that progress takes time and that there is no way to hurry the conditioning process, you will develop the patience to achieve Prime Triathlon. If you accept that you'll have setbacks in your training, you'll understand the need to persist in the face of this adversity.

Developing both patience and persistence will ensure that you stay positive and motivated long enough for the gains to occur and for you to achieve Prime Triathlon.

Patience means taking the time in training to develop your body along its timeline rather than along the timeline of your ego or logbook.
—Mark Allen

Seventh Law: Failure is necessary for Prime Triathlon. Many triathletes believe that failure, in the form of bad swims, rides, or runs, and poor results, is something to be avoided. But there can't be success without failure. Failure shows you what is not working. It means that you're moving out of your comfort zone and pushing yourself to new levels. Failure teaches you how to deal positively with adversity. Accepting failure as part of triathlon and learning the valuable lessons that failure can teach you will prepare you for the inevitable success that will follow.

Eighth Law: Prime preparation is devoted to readying you to perform your best under the most demanding conditions in the most important race of your life. We're not interested in you performing well in unimportant races, under ideal conditions, where you aren't faced with any adversity. The ultimate goal of Prime Triathlon is for you to perform your best when it really counts. Prime preparation will allow you to achieve Prime Triathlon in your equivalent of Hawaii Ironman®.

RECOVERY FROM TRAINING

Making rest and recovery a part of your training program is an indispensable contributor to your race preparations. Taking the time to recover is also, for many triathletes, a commitment that is difficult to adhere to because they worry that the time off will cause them to lose their fitness.

Building recovery into your training program serves several essential purposes. Contrary to what many triathletes believe, fitness gains aren't made when you work out. Your training efforts actually tear your body down. Periods of recovery allow your physical system to repair the damage and get stronger and more efficient. Rest days should be comprised of extra sleep, rejuvenating activities, such as massage, stretching, hot and cold baths, and rehydrating and refueling. Recovery also has important psychological bene-fits. Rest periods give you a break from the mental and emotional demands that training places on you. They give you time to reinvigorate your motiva-tion, intensity, focus, and enthusiasm that is depleted in training. Rest also helps you step back briefly from your training and allows you to maintain perspective and balance in how training fits into your life.

Scheduled recovery periods enable you to take minivacations from the intensity and monotony of training. These breaks allow you to replenish yourself physically and recharge your psychological and emotional batter-ies. Recovery should not be an optional part of your training program, but rather an absolute necessity for you to maximize your training and achieve your triathlon goals.

TAPERING

This chapter has been devoted to helping you get the most out of your training, getting you to be focused and intense, and helping you to main-tain your quality efforts. But the taper is one aspect of training we haven't discussed that is just as important as the hard work. Yet it strikes fear in the most seasoned triathlete. For the last several months leading up to an important race, you've been training your butt off getting ready for your big race. You've done everything you can in your training to have a successful race. You've been committed to your training program, missing few if any workouts and putting in your best effort in all aspects of your training.

Then, with your race approaching, you look at your training schedule and it reads, "Begin taper." You're faced with the pre-race taper, usually one week for an Olympic distance and up to three weeks for an Ironman. Like most triathletes, you might feel tightness in your chest and become short of breath. You start to get scared. You have crazy thoughts like, "I'm going to get out of shape. I'm going to get fat. If I back off now, there's no way I can have a good race." You're now experiencing "taper anxiety," the fear of losing everything you've gained from your training and failing to achieve your race goals.

Everyone talks about the importance of the taper and deep down you know you should commit to it. But each day that you go shorter distances with less intensity, you feel lazy. Taper anxiety can drive you to do crazy things—like a hard track workout or a long run a few days before your race. Jim saw extreme examples of taper anxiety when he arrived at Ironman® Lake Placid in 2002. One fellow he met rode the first loop of the bike—56 miles—three days before the race. A group of triathletes he knows went for a hilly, two-hour ride two days before the race.

When faced with taper anxiety, you're at a fork in the road that may determine whether or not you have a successful triathlon. If you give in to your taper anxiety and you maintain your training volume and intensity shortly before your race, you are almost guaranteed to fail to achieve your triathlon goals. You'll enter the race physically tired and mentally dull. You will lack strength, endurance, energy, motivation, confidence, and focus. You can expect to have a poor race. After your race you'll be angry at yourself for not following your program to the end. If you begin to take this fork in the road, be sure to have someone nearby who can talk some sense back into you. Having someone you trust who can help you regain your perspective and get you back on the road to tapering is essential.

It's simple; tapering will make your race. If you do a triathlon without a taper, you may bonk along the way or, at the very least, not perform up to your ability. Your body needs the taper to fully prepare itself for your race. The taper allows your body to rest, repairs all the damage, and maximizes the benefits you gained from the long, hard months of training.

I relish that downtime. You miss out a little bit when you're doing so much [training].

—Jeff Cuddleback, Ironman age-group world record holder

Because of its importance, it's critical to change your attitude toward the taper and relieve your taper anxiety. See it as an essential part of your training program that you must adhere to—would you skip workouts that are on your schedule? Enjoy this "chill" time before the race. See the taper as your reward for those last few weeks of high-volume, high-intensity training. Direct your energy into something else, such as spending more time with your family and friends, getting more things done at work, taking yoga, or getting a massage, anything that will either reduce your taper anxiety or at least distract you from it. Finally, tell yourself in no uncertain terms, "I must taper or I will not achieve my goals," believing that you will be rewarded for your commitment to the taper with a great race.

Preparing for a triathlon involves putting together all of the pieces of a complex puzzle—fitness, technique, equipment, tactics, and finally, the taper. Committing to a sufficient taper will not only ensure that you have the best race you are capable of and achieve your triathlon goals, but, more importantly, that you enjoy yourself every step of the way.

POST-RACE RECOVERY

Allowing yourself to recover adequately following a race is another essential part of a quality training program. Your willingness to recover fully from a race will affect how readily you're able to return to your season-long training program and direct your focus and energy into preparation for your next race. Yet much like tapering, post-race recovery can be a source of trepidation for triathletes, raising fears that they will lose their fitness and hinder their preparations for their next race.

The consequences of returning to a high-volume, high-intensity training program shortly after a race, particularly at longer distances, can be costly. In races that are physically demanding, microdamage to the muscles can occur that is not readily felt during day-to-day activities. It's not uncommon for triathletes to feel very good a few days after a race and assume they're recovered enough to get back to training. But when they go for a swim, bike, and particularly a run, the damage is felt. Returning too early aggravates whatever damage has been done in the race and slows the recovery process.

As I grow older I find I can't race as much. It is as mental as it is physical at this point. I have to really get up mentally to go out and put in a huge effort at a race. It takes me awhile to get mentally ready to race, and I find it harder trying to race events close together.

—Pete Kain

Post-race recovery is also necessary psychologically. You put a great deal of mental and emotional energy into your training and race preparations. Just like with physical effort, you need time to recover from the psychological wear and tear. Additionally, following the excitement of training and the race, some degree of post-race letdown is common, in which you may feel some sadness, a loss of motivation, and a lack of direction. This reaction is most pronounced when the race is unusually demanding or very important to you, and you're especially tired.

How long you should recover for following a race depends on a variety of factors. The longer the race, the more time you should take. Sprint and Olympic-distance races may only require a few days to recover, while for Ironman races, up to a month of recovery is typically recommended before a return to intense training. Your level of fitness also affects the length of your recovery. If you're in top shape and your body is accustomed to the demands of racing, then a shorter recovery can be expected. But if you're not in top shape or you're new to triathlon, you should allow more time to recover. The effort you expend in the race also influences the amount of recovery needed. It's possible to complete a triathlon, particularly shorter races, at a pace that places few demands on your body, meaning that little damage is done and only a short recovery is required. If, however, you raced the triathlon, that is, you competed to see how fast you could go and you pushed your body to its limits, you can expect considerable physical damage and an extended recovery will be needed.

Recovery doesn't mean lying on your couch for an extended period. Exercise physiologists recommend that, after anywhere from one to five days of complete rest, active rest not only encourages recovery, but also begins to prepare you for your return to training. Active rest involves doing light and noninvasive forms of exercise, for example, walking, easy spinning on an indoor trainer, and water running. These activities allow you to keep your muscles active while placing few demands on them.

I really suffered [in the 2000 Ironman® World Championships] and part of me doesn't want to ever go through that pain again. I thought if I trained harder than I had ever trained in the past that I would never suffer again in a race because I would be so far ahead of my competition. Well, that led to a year of overtraining and not having any strength during my races in 2001. This year I held back a lot during training sessions because I did not want to get into that overtraining mode.

—Peter Reid

OVERTRAINING

We have found that, as a general rule, triathletes are a highly motivated group. Rarely do triathletes come to us because they aren't training enough. More often, they're struggling because they're training too much. Overtraining is so common among triathletes because there are many different aspects of triathlon that require time, effort, and physical exertion. Combine this training load with high motivation—and often an obsessive personality—and you have a breeding ground for overtraining. Research has found that 20–25 percent of endurance athletes suffer from overtraining.

Overtraining can be caused by several factors. Training that involves too much volume or intensity with too high frequency can cause the body to break down and lead to overtraining. Declines in endurance, strength, and flexibility are common indications. Research has shown that overtraining is most often the result of a lack of adequate recovery from training volume and intensity. High volume and intensity are not inherently unhealthy, but they become so when you don't provide sufficient time for your body to repair itself and build on the physical damage that is incurred.

Symptoms of Overtraining

The experience of overtraining emerges subtly at first and then blossoms into a full-blown threat to your training and competitive pursuits. Your goal is to recognize the early signs of overtraining and respond to them appropriately before overtraining sets in and seriously interferes with your triathlon efforts. Overtraining presents you with a number of physical and psychological indicators to take note of. Physical symptoms related to overtraining include low energy, prolonged muscle fatigue and soreness, difficulty increasing training intensity, high heart rate or difficulty raising heart rate to normal training

Low motivation for me comes when I've been training too much. It's a sign to me that I need to back off. It's important to listen to that and look forward to some downtime to recharge.

—Victor Plata

levels, and slow recovery from previous workouts. More general physical symptoms consist of lethargy, persistent tiredness, lingering illness or injury, and difficulty sleeping. Psychological warning signs related to overtraining include a loss of motivation to train, decline in confidence, lack of direction, difficulty focusing, and reduced pain tolerance. General psychological indicators are depression, irritability, negative thinking, and loss of interest in other aspects of your life.

Contributors to Overtraining

A number of practical, physical, psychological, and social factors contribute to the emergence of overtraining. Being aware of these contributors while training can help identify their influence and keep them from pushing you to overtrain.

Practical. The substance and structure of your training program and race schedule can make you vulnerable to overtraining. A training program that schedules too many high-volume or high-intensity workouts each week will place physical demands on you that can lead to overtraining. For example, more than one high-intensity workout per week in each of the three disciplines is usually discouraged for all but the highest-level triathlete. A training program that doesn't provide adequate recovery also sets the stage for overtraining. Without sufficient rest after daily workouts, weekly schedules, and high-volume/high-intensity training periods, your body will not have enough time to heal and recover. Increasing training loads too quickly, in terms of frequency, volume, and intensity of workouts, without allowing your body to gradually adjust can cause overtraining. A competitive schedule that has too many races without sufficient time to recover can also result in overtraining.

Physical. Physical factors can contribute to overtraining. Minor illness and lingering injuries can exacerbate your vulnerability to overtraining by adding to the other already significant demands you place on your body in training. Poor nutrition, before, during, and after training, can cause your body to lack the nutrients necessary to effectively sustain the workload of your training schedule. Without proper fueling and hydration in all phases of training, your body will be unable to maintain itself and overtraining will be the likely result. Inadequate sleep is another physical contributor to overtraining. Because sleep is essential for your body to repair and recharge itself, too few hours or poor-quality sleep can prevent your body from getting the recovery time it needs to counter the demands of your training program. Life stress unrelated to your triathlon training can contribute to overtraining. Stress that you experience at work and home can place an undue burden above and beyond the demands that come from your training.

Mental. Overtraining can also be aggravated by psychological and emotional issues that drive you to train too hard or prevent you from getting adequate rest. An overinvestment in triathlon, in which you base your self-esteem on how you perform, can lead you to train excessively. The need for validation of your self-worth by meeting increasingly higher expectations in your training efforts and race results can cause you to ignore reason from coaches and training partners, and signals from your own body that it is breaking down under the strain. Specific psychological areas that affect this investment include perfectionism, insecurity, fear of failure, and self-criticism (see Chapter 16 for more on these issues). Additionally, qualities that are admired—dare we say worshipped—in triathletes, such as dedication, hard work, discipline, focus, intensity, and pain tolerance, when taken to the extreme, can impel you to overtrain.

If you're at all serious about your triathlon efforts, you're probably always looking for new ways to improve your fitness. Many triathletes are seduced by the classic American mentality that more is better; for example, if a 40-mile ride will improve your fitness, then you will have even more gains with a 60-mile ride. But a key lesson in triathlon is that more is not better and there are diminishing returns as you increase your volume and intensity. The more-is-better attitude will lead you directly to overtraining.

Social. If you train with others, you may feel pressure to keep up with them even when such a pace is harmful to you. This pressure is particularly noticeable during group rides and runs in which you may be highly motivated to stay with the group for self-esteem and social-acceptance reasons. In these situations, it's easy to raise your level of exertion—and go anaerobic—and rationalize it as being good for you. Though short periods of this intense effort won't do any harm, continued exertion outside your aerobic range will take its toll and lead to overtraining.

Recognizing warning signs

Many triathletes simply don't recognize the warning signs of overtraining. As we just described, overtraining has a clear set of physical and psychological symptoms. Unfortunately, these signs are often subtle or less noticeable individually. You may be so zealous or focused on your training that you don't notice them or you rationalize them as temporary states that you won't feel the next day. Only after the many symptoms have accumulated and overtraining has entrenched itself might you take notice and realize that you're overtrained. Another common reaction is to recognize them but be unwilling to respond to them. You may convince yourself that you can train through the symptoms or you may be loath to respond because to do so would be an admission of weakness.

Preventing Overtraining

The best way to deal with overtraining is to prevent it from occurring. You can take a number of practical, physical, and psychological steps to ensure that you strike a balance between training intensely enough to achieve your triathlon goals and allowing yourself to recover sufficiently so that you can continue your progress toward your training and competitive goals.

Understanding training. Prevention of overtraining starts with an understanding of triathlon training, the demands it can place on you, and how that knowledge can be translated into a quality training program. Buying into the notion that you should train smart, not hard, is the foundation for a sound training program. Effective training involves a periodized program of varied degrees of frequency, volume, and intensity in training accompanied by appropriate amounts of rest and recovery that will help you to progressively achieve your triathlon goals. A solid training program also includes specific training strategies that are fun, motivating, and that keep you mentally and emotionally fresh to help you avoid the monotony and routine that can set in during a long season.

Is it [low motivation] because I am overtrained? This is quite often the case when the motivation goes. The two are very connected—the mental aspect or motivation factor and the training state. If this is the case, then some easy training or time off to recharge the batteries is in order.

—Heather Fuhr

Confidence in your training program. One of the biggest causes of overtraining is when triathletes lose faith in their programs and decide to increase the volume and intensity. If you trust that your program will give you the results you want, you're more likely to adhere to the plan, particularly when you feel a pull to increase your efforts due to slow progress or seeing others improve faster than you are. Have confidence and patience with your program. Patience is often difficult in our microwave, fast-food, instant-coffee culture. Like everything of value in life, you will achieve your triathlon goals by allowing yourself the time needed to see the results you want.

Hydration and nutrition. You can reduce the risk of overtraining by ensuring that you fuel adequately for the demands you're placing on your body. You should have a healthy and balanced diet that provides you with the proper nutrients and sufficient calories to satisfy your training load.

Pre-, during, and post-workout nutrition that includes both solid food and hydration can also protect you from overtraining by ensuring that your body is well fueled for the burden you place on it.

Sleep. Getting enough sleep is also important for preventing overtraining. The more frequently and intensely you train, the more time your body needs to recover and repair itself. Shortchanging your body on this essential time of rest increases the chances of overtraining dramatically. Ensuring that you get plenty of sleep at night and take naps when needed during the day is some of the best preventive measures you can take.

Listening to your body. Listening to your body lies at the heart of preventing overtraining and is at once the most obvious and least followed lesson triathletes need to learn to keep from becoming overtrained. Your body communicates with you constantly about how it is responding to training, with heart rate, respiration, fatigue, pain, illness, and injury. Your body's messages are particularly loud when it's breaking down due to the volume and intensity of your training or lack of recovery time. Recognize these warning signs and act in your long-term best interests by adjusting your training in a way that will alleviate these early symptoms of overtraining.

Life stress. Interestingly, one of the most common causes of overtraining has nothing to do with triathlon training. Unless you're a pro triathlete whose life is devoted exclusively to the sport, you probably have a career, family, and other commitments that place considerable demands on your time and energy. Your "real world" can cause life stress that can wear your body down without even adding triathlon to the equation. You should factor these life stressors into your training program, then monitor and respond to them so that your life stress doesn't take its toll and interfere with your triathlon efforts.

Mental contributors. Psychological and emotional factors are more subtle, yet no less influential, contributors to overtraining. These mental issues are often what drive triathletes to train too often and too intensely, and don't allow them adequate time to recover. As we mentioned earlier (and will discuss in greater depth in Chapter 16), concerns such as overinvestment in triathlon, perfectionism, insecurity, life imbalance, social pressure, and unrealistic expectations can cause you to make poor decisions in your training that can lead to overtraining. Stepping back from, gaining perspective on, and exploring these areas can ensure that you aren't driven to overtrain by these unhealthy influences and that your attitude and emotions make a healthy contribution to your triathlon participation.

TRIATHLETE SPOTLIGHT: ELISA

Elisa was a self-admitted wimp when it came to training. At age 31, she liked doing triathlons, but wasn't much for training. She rarely gave her best effort and often gave up when faced with difficult conditions. This reaction frustrated her because she wasn't improving in her races. Also, her wimpiness didn't jibe with the drive and toughness that she exhibited in her career as a sales professional. Playing amateur shrink, she figured the reason it didn't carry over to her sports pursuits is because she had been a lousy athlete as a child and still thought of herself as very unathletic. Regardless, she was finally fed up enough to do something about it. She committed herself to toughening up and getting the most out of her training.

Once she made her commitment, she laid down some ground rules for herself. First, she would give her best effort in every workout. Second, she would keep going even when it hurt. Third, she would seek out tough conditions. Finally, she would not allow herself to quit no matter how much she might want to.

Before each training session, Elisa figured out what she wanted to accomplish and kept that focus in her mind through the workout. Also, rather than chatting with other members of her tri-club, she kept telling herself to "keep pushing" and "stay tough." Every time it started to get hard and she felt like quitting, she reminded herself of her commitment and kept going. On rainy or cold days, she forced herself to ride or run. And under no circumstances did she allow herself to give up.

At first, Elisa regretted her commitment. Training was so much harder and it hurt a lot more. But after a few weeks, hard training didn't seem quite so hard. The pain she felt during workouts wasn't quite so painful. She also noticed how happy she was after workouts compared to the disappointment she used to feel. She started to get excited when she looked out her window and saw a lousy day. She was feeling more confident, even tough. In her first race since her decision, she surprised herself with a big improvement over the previous year's race. More importantly, though, she kept pushing herself even when faced with a strong headwind in the last few miles of the run. After her race, Elisa realized something amazing: She had become one tough triathlete.

CHAPTER

11 Routines

R outines are critical tools for improving your training and race performances. Routines enable you to be completely physically, technically, tactically, and mentally prepared to perform your best. Most
triathletes use routines before races to make sure that they're prepared to have a great race. But routines can be used in other parts of your
training and races to further your triathlon goals. Routines can be developed in training to get the most out of a workout, for example, having a
good warm-up or making sure you get enough fuel during long rides.
Routines can also ensure your transitions are smooth, fast, and problem
free. We don't know a world-class or professional athlete in any sport who
doesn't use routines in some part of his or her competitive preparations.

There are many things that you can't control in your triathlon pursuits, for example, weather and course conditions. But there are some
things that you can control and routines can increase control over those
areas, such as your training and race readiness, by enabling you to prepare every area that influences your efforts. Areas you can control
include your equipment (is your bike in optimal condition?), your body
(are you physically warmed up and well fueled?), and your mind (are
you confident and focused?).

Routines also allow your preparations to be more predictable by ensuring that you're systematically covering every area that will influence performance. You can also plan for every eventuality that could arise during
a race. If you can reduce the things that can go wrong and are prepared

for those things that do, you'll be better able to stay focused and relaxed before and during the race.

All of your preparations involve a consistent narrowing of effort, energy, and focus. Each step closer to your training or race performances can lead you to that unique state of readiness in which you're physically and mentally capable of achieving your triathlon goals. Think of your preparation as a Prime Triathlon funnel (see below). Whatever you put into the funnel will dictate what comes out. If you put sound preparation into the funnel, what will come out is a successful performance.

I wanted to eliminate as many logistics issues as possible by being hyper prepared in my pre-race routine. That ensured that my full mind was there to race and nothing else got in the way.

—Mike Pigg

ROUTINES VS. RITUALS

Some sport psychologists use the term "ritual" in place of routine. We don't like "ritual," though, because of the negative connotations it carries. A ritual

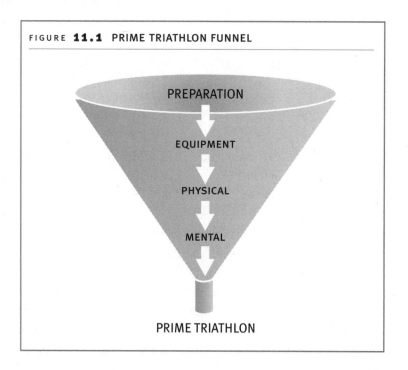

FIGURE **11.1** PRIME TRIATHLON FUNNEL

PREPARATION

EQUIPMENT

PHYSICAL

MENTAL

PRIME TRIATHLON

is associated with superstitions and is often made up of things that have no practical impact on performance, such as wearing lucky socks or following a specific route to the race site. Routines are only composed of practices that have a direct impact on performance. Rituals are rigid and ceremonial. You may believe that rituals must be done or you won't perform well, even when the rituals have no real influence over your performances. Routines, on the other hand, can be adjusted should the need arise; for example, if you arrive late to a race, you can shorten your routine and still get prepared. The key distinction is that you control routines, but rituals control you.

Remember that the goal of routines is to totally prepare you for training and races. Everything done in a routine serves a specific and practical function in that readiness process, for example, a physical and technical warm-up and a review of tactics for an upcoming race.

Benefits of Routines

Routines have many benefits for training and racing. Foremost, they develop consistency in all areas that affect your triathlon efforts. Consistency in your preparations leads to consistent thinking, intensity, focus, emotions, and physical and technical readiness. By consistently going through a routine, you're training your mind and body to respond the same way regardless of the situation. Routines are also flexible and can be adjusted to different situations that arise, for example, a delay in the start of the race. Flexibility in your routine means you won't be surprised or stressed by changes that occur during your preparations and you're less likely to be affected by race pressure. Routines enable you to perform your best in a wider range of situations and conditions.

Routines have great benefits psychologically. They build your confidence because you're more comfortable and in control, and each step of your routine tells you that you're doing everything you need to be successful. They help you achieve ideal intensity that will maximize your triathlon efforts. You'll feel relaxed, but energized and strong and physically ready to race. By progressing through your routine, you mobilize your body to the level of intensity that enables it to be most efficient in the race. A routine also enables you to focus on those areas that will help you perform well. Focusing on your routine also keeps your mind away from distractions and negativity that could hurt your performance.

Regardless of whether you're preparing for a low-key race at the start of the season or the most important race of the year, routines signal to you that this is just another race for which you'll be ready. Ultimately, the goal of routines in training and races is to ensure that when you start your race, you're totally physically, technically, tactically, and mentally prepared to perform your best.

Training Routines

A training routine helps you get physically and mentally prepared to gain the most benefit from your efforts. Training routines also give you experience in using routines so when you use them before races and in transitions, you'll be comfortable and able to gain the same benefits. For you to get the most out of your workouts, develop a brief training routine that ensures that you're totally prepared for every effort. These training routines are most useful for your quality workouts when you need to be focused and intense to maximize their value. Training routines are less important for longer workouts at lower intensity because quality is not the emphasis.

The first step in your training routine is getting your body ready. This involves checking and adjusting your intensity as needed and warming up and stretching so your body is primed for a quality workout. This part of your training routine could include deep breathing to relax yourself for a set of swim drills or using intense breaths and jumping up and down to raise your intensity for 800-meter intervals on the track. Second, distractions and a lack of focus are common causes of poor-quality training. We often see triathletes before they begin a workout chatting with others or looking around rather than focusing on what they need to get the most out of their efforts. Shortly before you begin a workout, focus on its purpose. Know and focus on precisely what you want to accomplish in the workout and what you need to achieve that goal, for example, focus on technique or effort. The techniques we described in Chapter 6—for example, controlling your eyes, repeating keywords, and maintaining a relaxed body—can help you find that focus, so as the workout begins, your body and mind are ready to gain the benefits from your efforts. Your training routine need only last a few seconds, but will completely prepare you to get the most out of your training. It will also lay the foundation for pre-race and transition routines.

Pre-race Routines

The next step in developing effective routines is to create a pre-race routine that is an extended version of the training routine. The goal is the same, to be totally prepared to perform your best, but the difference is that the purpose of a pre-race routine is to prepare you for a longer and more intense and demanding event, and it can take several hours to complete.

There isn't one ideal routine for every triathlete but all have common elements. You have to decide what exactly to put into your routine and how to structure it. Developing an effective pre-race routine is a progressive process; it will take time to find one that works for you. There are a variety of practical, physical, and psychological concerns that you must consider in developing your pre-race routine.

Equipment Preparation and Organization

Triathlon is a complicated sport that requires many pieces of equipment—wet suit and goggles, bike and helmet, and running shoes—in addition to an assortment of essential accessories: sunscreen, sunglasses, water bottles, gels, energy bars, and spare tubes, just to name a few. The likelihood of something being forgotten or going wrong with all of this gear is more the rule than the exception. You can minimize the chances of a problem arising by addressing the preparation and organization of your equipment and the myriad accessories in your pre-race routine. In developing your pre-race routine, know the what, where, and how for making sure all of your gear is ready to go and where it needs to be at the right time. We've provided a list of items you may need for your triathlon (see Triathlon

I'd sit in my hotel or condo watching the sun come up, thinking about my race at 5:00 in the morning the week before a race. I'd do that every morning. I'd visualize what was going to happen, what I would do when I got up, what I was going to eat, what time I was going to head down to the race. I'd always take a shower before the race, drink a cup of hot tea, all the clothes laid out so I didn't have to take energy away from my race. I wanted it to be methodical. I wanted that stuff to be intuitive so that I could think more about my competitors or my race rather than the logistics issues. Before and during the race, I'd think about transitions, "Goggles down, sunglasses on, helmet on, boom boom boom." No more thought than that. Keeping it simple was important. I never felt like there were chinks in the armor before races. With logistics second nature, once the gun went off, all I had to do was my best.

—Mike Pigg

Preparation List on page 161) and a list of transition area gear and preparation you need to do before your race (see Transition Area Gear and Preparation on page 162).

Physical Preparation

Your pre-race routine can ensure that every contributor to your physical preparation is addressed at the proper time in the best possible way. Foremost among the physical concerns is your pre-race fueling. Eat a nutritious breakfast of familiar foods two to three hours before your event and perhaps have a gel or banana shortly before the race to allow for timely digestion and access to energy. Also hydrate properly before your race. And don't forget to go to the bathroom as needed. Having a clear and settled digestive system can be a make-or-break factor in a race. A good physical warm-up, which might include a short run, stretch, or swim, also helps prepare your body for your race. Know what will physically prepare you for your race and when and where your warm-up will occur.

Focus Needs

If you have an internal focus style, the goal in your pre-race routine is to put yourself in a place where there are few external distractions and where you can focus on your pre-race preparations. To maintain that narrow Mag-Lite® beam, go through your pre-race routine away from other people and activities that could distract you.

If you have an external focus style, the goal in your pre-race routine is to put yourself in a place where you're unable to become focused internally and think about the race excessively. An external focus style means that you need to keep your Mag-Lite® beam wide during your preparations so you can keep your mind off the upcoming race and away from thinking too much. Your pre-race routine should be done where there is enough activity to draw your focus away from inside your head. To widen the beam, go through your pre-race routine around people and activities that can draw your focus outward.

Intensity Needs

You'll also want to build your pre-race routine around your intensity needs. The intensity component of your pre-race routine includes checking your intensity periodically before the start of the race and using psych-up or psych-down techniques to adjust it as needed. Set aside time in your

TRIATHLON PREPARATION LIST

BIKE

1. Bike
2. Shoes
3. Helmet
4. Tubes (2) and tires
5. Pump
6. CO_2
7. Bike stand
8. Tool bag
   a. tape (electric, duct)
   b. flat-repair kit
   c. chain oil

CLOTHING

1. Swim
   a. wet suit
   b. lid
   c. goggles (2 pair)
   d. defog fluid
   e. earplugs
2. Bike
   a. tri-outfit (top and shorts)
   b. socks
   c. gloves
   d. sunglasses
      (light and dark lenses)
3. Run
   a. socks
   b. hat
   c. baby powder
   d. shoe horn
   e. water-bottle waist pack or
      Fuel Belt
4. General
   a. heart rate monitor
   b. number belt

CLOTHING (continued)

   c. towels (2 small and 2 large)
   d. water bottles
      (aero, 2 tall, 3 small)
   e. extra laces

FUEL

1. Endurance and recovery powder
2. Food
3. Gels
4. Salt or electrolyte tablets

PRE- AND POST-RACE CLOTHING, FUEL, AND SUNDRIES

1. T-shirt
2. Long-sleeve shirt
3. Shorts
4. Warm-up pants
5. Sandals
6. Dry socks
7. Hat
8. Garbage bag for wet suit
9. Dirty-laundry bag
10. Hydration
11. Food

MEDICAL KIT

1. Body Glide
2. Sunscreen
3. Band-aids
4. Chapstick
5. Vasoline
6. Baby powder
7. Aspirin and anti-inflammatories
8. Athletic tape
9. Shaver

TRANSITION AREA GEAR AND PREPARATION

TRANSITION GEAR	TRANSITION PREP
1. Bike	1. Load fuel-bars, gel, liquids on bike.
2. Towels (small and large)	
3. Water bottle for rinsing feet	2. Lay out transition.
4. Tri-top	3. Roll and powder socks.
5. Helmet (gloves and glasses inside)	4. Powder running shoes.
	5. Put on race belt.
6. Cycling shoes and socks (powdered and rolled)	6. Put on sunscreen.
	7. Check tires.
7. Number belt	8. Correct gear on the bike.
8. Running shoes, socks, and shoe horn	9. Put on heart rate monitor.
9. Running hat	
10. Gels (place in pocket)	
11. Salt or electrolyte tabs (place in pocket)	

routine when you can use these strategies. As you approach the race, move closer to your prime intensity. The short period just before the swim start should be devoted to a final check and adjustment of your intensity.

If you perform best at a lower level of intensity, you want your pre-race routine to be done at a leisurely pace and allow plenty of opportunity to take breaks to slow down and relax. Be around people who are relaxed and low-key as well. If you race best at a higher level of intensity, your pre-race routine can be done at a faster pace with more energy put into the components of your routine. Make sure that you're constantly doing something. There should be little time during which you're just standing around and waiting. You'll want to be around people who are energetic and outgoing.

A part of addressing your intensity needs involves being aware of how much stress you feel on the morning of the race. If you tend to get nervous before races, recognize when the stress becomes a problem, either emotionally or physically, and have strategies, such as deep breathing or muscle relaxation, built into your pre-race routine to relieve the stress.

Designing a Pre-race Routine

Designing a pre-race routine that will optimally prepare you for your race helps ensure that you achieve your race goals. Creating a pre-race routine involves figuring out what you need to do, and where, when, and how you need to do everything to get ready for your race.

What. The first step in designing a pre-race routine is to make a list of everything you need to do before a race to be prepared. Some of the common elements to include are meals, review of race tactics, physical warm-up, technical warm-up, equipment check, and mental preparation. Other more personal things that might go into a pre-race routine include going to the bathroom, putting on your race clothing and wet suit, and fueling just before the start. Because triathlon is so complex and there are so many different elements you must prepare for, a clear and detailed understanding of what you need to do is essential to ensure that you don't forget anything. A common practice for triathletes, and an absolute necessity for longer-distance races, is to prepare a list of everything you need to have and to do the morning of a race (see page 161 and 162).

Then, decide in what order you want to execute the components of your list as you approach the start of the race. In figuring out the order of your pre-race routine, consider the race setting and activities, such as access to a kitchen for breakfast, distance to the start from your accommodations, and transition layout.

Where. Next, specify where each step of your routine can best be completed by using your knowledge of the race venue and transition areas. Surveying the race site the day before can help you identify where you can best accomplish each aspect of your pre-race routine. If you're a first timer at a race, don't be shy about asking race officials and veteran competitors to help you get "the lay of the land." Getting to know T1 and the swim-start area is particularly useful as you address your focus and intensity needs; for example, if you like to be alone before a race, is there a quiet place where you can get away from other competitors?

I do an easy warm-up [before a race]. I am pretty relaxed about racing, so I'm usually one of the last people there. Most of my friends don't like going with me to a race since I like to sleep in and just get there before the start.

—Pete Kain

When. Finally, establish a time frame and a schedule for completing your pre-race routine. In other words, what time do you want to wake up and how much time do you need to get totally prepared? For example, at shorter distances, triathletes typically like to eat 75 to 120 minutes before they race. In contrast, for Ironman races, most competitors like to eat 150 to 200 minutes before the race. Also, some triathletes like to get to T1 hours before the race. Others like to arrive only a short time before. All of these decisions are personal. Find out what works best for you. Use the Personalized Pre-race Routine form on page 165 to assist you in developing your pre-race routine.

How. Once your pre-race routine is organized, try it out at some less-important races (Warning: Never try a new routine at your most important race of the season!). Some things may work and others may not. In time, you'll be able to fine-tune your routine until you find the one that's most comfortable and best prepares you for a race. Lastly, remember, pre-race routines only have value if you use them consistently. If you use your routine before every race, in a short time, you won't even have to think about doing it. Your pre-race routine will simply be what you do before each race, and it will ensure that you're totally prepared to perform your best.

It's important to think where you want your mind-set to be when you arrive at the transition area in the morning. There can be a lot of tension in the air. Make a commitment to staying in your mental zone.

—Lance Watson, triathlon coach

Who. Depending on your focus style, you will either prefer to be alone or with others leading up to your race. Decide ahead of time if you will be traveling to the race with other people—for example, training partners, family, friends—or alone. If you go with others, ask yourself if they are people with whom you will feel relaxed and comfortable, who will respect your focus and intensity needs, and whether they will hamper or bolster your preparations and allow you to adhere to your pre-race routine. Communicate your needs (and ask them theirs) before the trip so there will be no confusion or conflict.

Transition Routines

Transitions are the most neglected aspects of triathlons. Transitions are like the crazy uncle of triathlon; everyone in the family knows that he's there and they know he can wreck the family holiday, but every family

PERSONALIZED PRE-RACE ROUTINE FORM

Directions: List the pre-race activities that will help you totally prepare to perform your best.

EARLY-MORNING

1. Nutrition:

2. Equipment:

3. Physical:

4. Mental:

ARRIVAL AT T1

1. Nutrition:

2. Equipment:

3. Physical:

4. Mental:

FINAL PREPARATION

1. Nutrition:

2. Equipment:

3. Physical:

4. Mental:

member is so busy getting the party ready and having a good time that he's forgotten until he drops the Christmas turkey or Easter ham. Yet any veteran triathlete will tell you that transitions can make or break a race. T1 and T2 can be brief, smooth, and calming shifts from swim to bike or bike to run. Or they can be interminable purgatories of stress, distraction, and confusion. Which ones they are for you depends on whether you have a transition routine to guide you through them. You can set yourself up to arrive at your transition either cool, calm, and collected, or tired, out of breath, and stressed. Take control of your transitions to be sure that you move to the next stage of the race as effortlessly and quickly as possible.

Your transition area

The first key to a quality transition is a well-organized transition area. The transition is a zone of frenetic activity in which gear is dropped, donned in the wrong order, or just plain forgotten. To prevent confusion and chaos in your transitions, know where everything is and in what order you will address each piece of gear without having to think about it. Create a practice transition area at home weeks before your race and memorize where you place, in T1, your towel, bike socks and shoes, sunglasses, and helmet, and, in T2, your running socks and shoes, hat, and gels (and whatever else you like to have in your transition areas). Visualize this process in your training so that it becomes second nature.

Your transition area layout should have a logical arrangement. Place your transition gear based on the order in which you will need it and its accessibility at the right point in your transition. What will you need to do when you first arrive at T1 (e.g., strip off your wet suit)? What order will you then proceed through T1 (e.g., dry feet with towel, put on socks and cycling shoes, put on sunglasses and helmet, unrack your bike)? Your answers to these questions will determine where you place your transition items next to your bike. You will ask similar questions for your T2 transition. In most races, the two transitions are one and the same (except for point-to-point triathlons), so a further challenge is the placement of your T1 and T2 gear in a very limited space. Also, remove from the transition area all of the gear and clothing that you will not be using during the race. If you don't have an alternate location for these items while you're racing, stow it in your gear bag or backpack and place it in the back of your transition area out of the way of your race gear. Clearing your transition area of unnecessary clutter will minimize confusion and make your transitions smoother.

Your transition process

The second key is to have a well-learned transition process. When you lay out your transitions at home before the race, practice your transitions until you can do them quickly, smoothly, and without confusion or mistakes. Try to race through it as fast as possible to simulate the hectic pace of a real transition. Once you have a problem-free practice transition down, do it a few more times to really ingrain your transition routine because, in the race, you won't be as composed and relaxed.

Five-step transition routine

In addition to the logistics of your transitions, you also have to deal with the psychology and physiology of transitions. You can take active steps to ensure that your mind and body are ready to segue from swim to bike and bike to run as smoothly and with as little disruption as possible. We recommend the Five R's, a five-step transition routine.

Ready. Transition routines actually start before you arrive at T1 and T2. In the 100 yards before you emerge from the water, you want to get yourself physically and mentally ready to have an efficient transition. You can slow your pace a bit and allow your heart rate to settle down. If you're like many triathletes, you don't kick much during the swim to save your leg muscles. To increase circulation in your legs to prepare them for the sprint to your transition area, you can begin kicking more (but not necessarily harder). As you near the shore, you want to shift your focus from the swim to your transition. Remind yourself of the layout of your transition area and review your transition routine so you have fresh in your mind where everything is, the first thing you will do, and what exactly will follow.

In the last half mile of your bike before you arrive at T2, you similarly want to prepare yourself physically and mentally for your transition to the run. As you approach T2, take stock of how your body feels and decide what you want to do physically. Slow your cadence, stretch your legs, eat a gel, or take in extra fluids. Also refocus on the transition and get ready mentally, as for T1, by reminding yourself of your transition layout and routine.

For both T1 and T2, the pace that you run (or walk) to your transition area will depend on its distance and terrain and how tired and out of breath you are. Remember that the few seconds you gain from a mad sprint to your transition area may not be worth the physical price you pay for the increased exertion. This transition-within-a-transition is a good place to settle down and prepare yourself for your transition routine when you arrive at your transition.

Recovery. As you leave the water or get off your bike and enter the transition area, allow your body to rest, however briefly. The recovery phase of your transitions emphasizes taking several slow, deep breaths and encouraging your heart rate to slow in anticipation of the start of the next leg of your race. If you can lower your heart rate ten beats per minute during your transition, you'll gain a significant recovery benefit between each leg of the race. This is especially important after a long or demanding swim or bike in which you become fatigued and out of breath. Deep breathing and relaxing your muscles also help you focus and better prepare you for the next R.

Regroup. This phase of your transition routine addresses your emotions at that point in the race. Particularly when your race hasn't gone as well as planned, you may feel a variety of negative emotions, such as frustration, anger, or despair. Regrouping allows you to gain awareness of how you feel and how your emotions are affecting your motivation, confidence, and intensity. Use the transition as an opportunity to regroup and start the next leg of your race with a better frame of mind. Because of the powerful influence that emotions have, your ability to "get your act together" emotionally during transitions can help or hurt your race.

An important realization is that how you did in the previous legs of your race aren't necessarily related to how you will do the rest of the race. For example, a poor swim doesn't necessarily mean that you're in for a bad bike or run. But one thing that can connect each leg of a triathlon is the emotions that you carry across your transitions. If you're frustrated and angry coming into T1 or T2, you increase your chances of letting those emotions hurt the rest of your race. Conversely, if you're excited and happy about the previous leg of your race, you increase your chances of the remainder of your race going well. Using your transition to regroup will enable you to let go of the negative emotions and replace them with positive emotions that will help you finish on an upbeat note.

Refocus. Some triathletes have a tendency during races, especially when a race isn't going well, to focus on how poorly the swim or bike has gone. If this happens to you, return to a process focus for the next leg of your race. During the refocus phase of your transition routine, first evaluate how things have gone so far and how well your race tactics have worked. Then, focus on what you need to do so the rest of your race goes well. Your focus can be physical (e.g., staying relaxed), technical (e.g., maintaining a smooth cadence), tactical (e.g., staying in your aerobic range), or mental (e.g., staying positive and motivated). The important thing is to leave the transition area with a clear focus on what you want to do to improve a poor race or continue a good race.

Recharge. Just as transitions start before you arrive at T1 or T2, they also don't end when you leave the transition area. The first five to ten minutes of your bike or run should include an assessment of how your body feels and whether it's ready for this phase of the race. You can then decide what you need to do to prepare yourself physically for this leg of the race, for example, adjusting your technique and pace, relaxing your body, or fueling and hydrating.

Race Routines

There's an important place for routines during the race outside of transitions. Because triathlon is so complicated it's easy to forget to do important things during your race, for example, fueling, hydrating, and stretching. Particularly in longer races where the physical and psychological demands are great, forgetting to do some of these necessities can have dire consequences. Race routines, which will depend on the race distance, can include drinking every 15 minutes, changing your body position every 30 minutes, and eating every 20–30 minutes on the bike. On the run, your race routine can include swinging your arms and settling your shoulders every mile, drinking at every aid station, and having a gel every 2 miles. Race routines act as reminders of key contributors to your race, particularly late in races when you're tired and in pain and you may forget to do things that will help you finish.

TRIATHLETE SPOTLIGHT: DENNIS

If you looked at Dennis's life, you'd wonder how he got through the day. His house was a mess, his hair was unkempt, his clothes were wrinkled, his car was strewn with litter, and his office filing system consisted of piles of folders. But, oddly, his triathlon life was the only area of his life that seemed to have order and it ran like a well-oiled machine. At age 56, he relished the complexity of the sport and took immense pride in mastering all of its intricacies. He particularly enjoyed his pre-race preparation. He had his pre-race routine down to a science.

Two nights before the race, a half-Ironman distance, Dennis began by doing a complete inspection of his bike, cleaning and oiling his chain, tightening bolts, and testing his gears and brakes. He would then print out the preparation list he kept on his computer and lay out and pack all of his clothing and gear, checking and double checking each item as he stowed it in his travel bag. He would always eat the same pasta and salad dinner with one chocolate cookie.

Dennis was especially proud of his transitions. At the beginning of each season, in his backyard, he would test out the placement of his transition items and practice his transitions until he could do them with his eyes closed, literally. His local tri-club even asked him to give a transitions clinic to its members. The day before the race, he would reconnoiter the transition area, ensuring he knew exactly how to get in and out in the fastest possible time. He placed a piece of bright orange ribbon at the end of the row on which he racked his bike so he could find his bike quickly.

The night before the race, in his hotel room, Dennis laid out his race clothing, methodically prepared his energy drinks, taped his gels to the top tube of his bike, and packed his transition bag. He then went to a local Italian restaurant where he had made reservations and had the same dinner as the previous night.

On race morning, he woke up two hours before the start, ate his customary breakfast of half a bagel with peanut butter, a banana, a plain yogurt, and a glass of orange juice. He then went for a ten-minute jog to warm up his body, put on his race clothing, double checked his transition bag, pumped up his bike tires, and drove to the race, arriving sixty minutes before the start.

During the ensuing hour, Dennis laid out his well-organized transition area, went to the bathroom, put on his wet suit, and waited for his start wave. He always kept to himself before races, preferring to stay quiet, calm, and focused on his race.

After a good swim, as usual, his T1 went smoothly and he headed out on the bike. During the ride, he drank and fueled at predetermined intervals, and stretched every 5 miles. At about mile 35, he got a flat tire. He didn't panic though. Not surprisingly, he had a precise routine for flats, having practiced changing tubes dozens of times at home, and he was on his way again in less than five minutes.

Dennis's T2 went equally well and he began his run. He maintained a good pace throughout, taking in two cups of water at each aid station and eating a gel every thirty minutes. He finished strong and crossed the finish line satisfied with his well-organized and meticulously executed effort.

C H A P T E R

12 Mental Imagery

M ental imagery is a powerful, and often forgotten, tool for improving your training and race performances. It's used by virtually all great athletes in every sport and there's considerable scientific research supporting its value. Imagery is beneficial because it influences every contributor to Prime Triathlon. Imagery increases motivation by allowing you to see and feel yourself giving your best effort and reaching your goals. It builds confidence by enabling you to imagine yourself performing well and succeeding. Imagery improves intensity by allowing you to see and experience race stress and use psych-up or psych-down techniques to control it. It enhances focus by identifying important cues and letting you rehearse prime focus. Imagery enables you to generate positive emotions in response to seeing and feeling yourself perform your best. Finally, it can help you better manage your training and race pain by allowing you to practice pain-mastery techniques.

Imagery also improves technical, tactical, and race skills. It ingrains the image and feeling of correct technique and provides imagined repetition of proper execution. Imagery enables you to further learn sound tactics and to instill effective race skills, habits, and routines. Think of imagery as weight training for the mind. Much as strength training has numerous physical benefits, imagery can fortify many mental areas.

Many sport psychologists, coaches, and athletes use the term "visualization" to describe this tool. But visualization places too much emphasis on its visual component. The power of this technique lies well beyond its visual aspects. The most effective imagery involves the complete, multi-sensory reproduction of the actual triathlon experience.

Imagery can be used in several settings that will help you achieve Prime Triathlon. During training in which you're focusing on better technique, you can use it to enhance your technical skills and improve the quality of training. As part of your pre-race preparations, you can use imagery to rehearse key parts of your race and ingrain positive reactions to adversity to prime your intensity and focus.

> *It's a lot easier to go faster when you're in the right mind-set. Going through [mental imagery] is like getting free time.*
>
> —Mark Allen

IMAGERY IS A SKILL

Imagery is a skill, just like a technique, that develops with practice. Few athletes have ideal imagery when they first use it. It's common for those who haven't used imagery before to struggle with it initially. This may cause discouragement and lead to the belief that imagery can't be beneficial. But if you put in the time and effort, your imagery will improve and become a valuable tool.

The first thing to do is assess your imagery abilities. After reading the following imagery skills descriptions, complete the Imagery Skills Profile on page 178. This will give you a graphic representation of your imagery strengths and weaknesses. Then, use the exercise described with each imagery skill to strengthen the imagery skills you need to improve most.

Imagery Perspective

Imagery perspective refers to the location of the "imagery camera" when you do imagery. You can use one of two perspectives. The internal perspective involves seeing yourself from inside your body looking out as if you were actually performing. The imagery camera is inside your head looking out through your eyes. The external perspective involves seeing yourself from outside your body like on video. The imagery camera follows your performance from the outside. (1–all internal; 5–both; 10–all external)

Research indicates that one perspective isn't better than the other. Rather, most people have a dominant perspective with which they're most comfortable. There are also some people who are equally adept at both perspectives. You should use the perspective that's most natural for you and then experiment with the other perspective to see if it helps you in a different way.

Imagery Control

Have you ever been doing imagery and you can't stop yourself from doing poorly; for example, you keep seeing yourself sinking in the pool or you feel like you're towing a car on an imagined hill climb? This problem relates to imagery control, which is how well you're able to imagine what you want to imagine. Though it's not uncommon for athletes new to imagery to perform poorly in their imagery, this difficulty can be frustrating and puzzling.

Poor imagery control demonstrates the power of the unconscious mind. Imagery is guided by your unconscious beliefs. Most directly, imagery reflects your deepest beliefs about your ability to be successful. If you don't have confidence that you can swim, bike, or run well, your imagery won't be able to recreate good performances. Poor imagery control then tells you that you need to improve your confidence. Imagery is also a great tool for judging progress in developing your confidence. Improved imagery control is a sign of increased confidence at its deepest level.

Imagery control is a skill that develops with practice. If mistakes occur in your imagery, you shouldn't just let them go by. If you do, you'll ingrain the negative image and feeling, which will hurt your performances. Instead, when you perform poorly in your imagery, immediately rewind the "imagery video" and edit it. That is, rerun the imagery video until you do it correctly. (1–no control; 10–total control)

Visual Imagery

Visual imagery involves how clearly you see yourself performing. Ideally, your visual images should be as clear as if you are actually performing. It may be, though, that your images are blurry or you can't see yourself at all.

Knowing what you look like when swimming, biking, and running can help your visual imagery. Too often, triathletes don't know what they look like, so they imagine themselves performing like someone they train with or like a top triathlete. In either case, your imagery may not be most beneficial because you'll be seeing someone else rather than yourself perform. A video camcorder is a great tool for helping you develop clear and accurate images of how you swim, bike, and run. A few minutes of each part of triathlon is all you need to help you ingrain a proper image. You can also bolster your visual self-image by imagining yourself wearing your usual training and race clothing and using your own bike and other gear, and imagining yourself in familiar training or race settings, for example, where you usually swim, do bike hill repeats, or run track intervals. (1-unclear; 10-clear)

Auditory Imagery

Vivid auditory images are important because sounds can play an important role in your triathlon performances, for example, the sound of the water during a swim, the pounding of your feet during a run, or your breathing. Using the sounds of triathlon can deepen the imagery experience and facilitate its benefits. (1-unclear; 10-clear)

Physical Imagery

We believe that the most powerful part of imagery is feeling it in your body. This kinesthetic sense, for example, your swim stroke, cycling cadence, and running turnover, is what will deeply ingrain new technical and mental skills and habits. Also, your ability to feel pain in your imagery will help you to instill pain-mastery skills that will help you when you're actually training and racing. A useful way to increase the feeling in imagery is to combine imagined and real sensations. Imagine yourself performing and move your body with the imagined performance. By integrating the imagined sensations with the actual physical feelings, you can improve the value of your imagery even more. (1-unclear; 10-clear)

Thoughts

What you think during a race often dictates your motivation, confidence, intensity, focus, emotions, pain, and how you perform. Imagery gives you the ability to learn new and better ways of thinking during training and races. You can generate race situations in your imagery in which you've expressed negative self-talk and practice positive thinking in its place. Drawing on the techniques described in Chapter 4, you can replace the negative self-talk with positive expressions that will help you become your best ally. Using imagery in this way enables you to gain the added repetition of positive thinking that will further ingrain new positive thinking skills and enable you to more readily access them when needed even when you're away from training. (1-no thoughts; 10-usual thoughts)

Emotions

As Chapter 7 indicated, emotions play an important role in your ability to perform your best. Incorporating them into your imagery can be a valuable way to strengthen the positive influence emotions have on your performances and to ensure that you're capable of generating positive emotions when needed most. Much like in actual races, imagining scenarios that have in the past evoked negative emotions gives you the opportunity to respond to them in a more positive way. (1–no emotions; 10–strong emotions)

Total Image

Another key aspect of imagery is being able to imagine the total performance. The more you can completely recreate your training and race experiences, the more accurate, real, and beneficial the images will be. The most effective imagery reproduces every aspect of your actual triathlon performance, duplicating the sights, sounds, physical sensations, thoughts, and emotions that you would experience at an actual race. (1–poor reproduction; 10–exact reproduction)

Maximizing Imagery

To help you get the most out of your imagery, it's essential to fully develop your imagery skills. The exercises below were designed to help you do this. Remember that each of the imagery skills areas can be developed with practice.

- *Exercise 1: Imagery perspective.* Imagine yourself performing some aspect of triathlon twice for thirty seconds; for example, imagine doing laps in the pool. The first time use your dominant perspective. The next time use the other perspective. You may find that only one perspective works for you or that you can use either perspective equally well. In either case, for the time being, rely on the perspective that comes most naturally to you.

- *Exercise 2: Imagery control.* Imagine yourself performing five times for thirty seconds. In each segment, if you do poorly, rewind and edit your imagery until you get it right. We've sometimes found it difficult for triathletes to edit their imagery when they imagine themselves performing at full speed, for example, a 50-yard sprint in

IMAGERY SKILLS PROFILE

Directions: After reading each imagery description, indicate how you perceive yourself on a 1–10 scale for each factor by referring to the text on page 174. Complete the profile by drawing a line at that rating number and shading in the area toward the center of the profile. Before rating yourself on each factor, close your eyes and imagine performing for thirty seconds, paying attention to a particular factor. Except for the perspective factor, a score below 7 indicates an area in need of improvement.

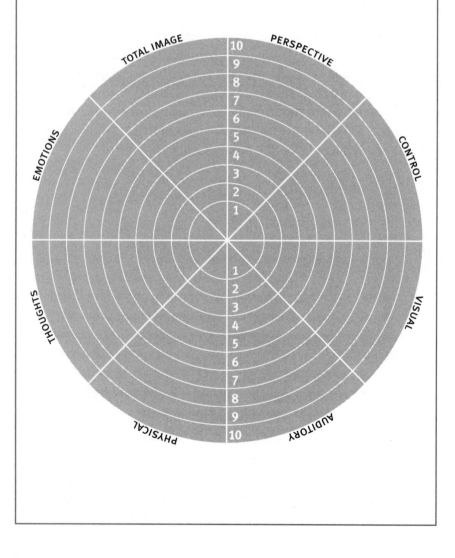

the pool. It can be helpful when you're having difficulty controlling your imagery to slow it down, in which you see and feel yourself performing in slow motion, even frame by frame. This technique enables you to have greater control of your imagery. As you gain imagery control in slow motion, you can progressively increase the speed of your imagery while maintaining good control until you're able to perform well at "real time" speed.

- *Exercise 3: Visual imagery.* Watch yourself performing on video, then immediately close your eyes and reproduce the video images. As the visual image of how you perform becomes clearer, put away the video for a while and repeat the accurate visual images of your performances. If the image starts to fade, return to the video until you're able to see yourself performing consistently. This exercise will help you ingrain an accurate image of how you perform.

- *Exercise 4: Auditory imagery.* Imagine performing three times for thirty seconds. Each time, focus on a different sound associated with your performance. Once you're able to do this consistently, put all of the sounds together and hear the various sounds in one sequence of imagery.

- *Exercise 5: Physical imagery.* Imagine performing an aspect of triathlon two times for thirty seconds. Each time, focus on feeling your muscles and the physical movements. Then, imagine performing two more times focusing on the feeling, but this time, move your body with the imagery to simulate the actual movement. Obviously, it's not possible to physically simulate the complete movements of swimming, biking, or running while lying down. But you can move your hands in small motions that can approximate the swim stroke, pedal stroke, and running stride. You may also find that the rest of your body starts to move of its own accord. By combining the imagined feelings with the actual physical feelings, you'll further enhance the quality of imagery and increase its benefits.

- *Exercise 6: Thoughts.* Imagine yourself in a difficult race situation, for example, riding into a headwind, where you've used negative self-talk in the past. Allow yourself to experience the negative thoughts, then imagine replacing the negatives with positive self-talk. Follow the positive self-talk with imagining yourself performing better with more motivation and confidence.

- **Exercise 7: Emotions.** Imagine yourself in an emotionally challenging race situation, for example, starting to get frustrated from the physical contact and rough water during the mass start of a swim. Allow yourself to experience the frustration and then replace the negative emotions with positive ones, such as calm and resolve.

- **Exercise 8: Total image.** Imagine yourself performing five times for thirty seconds. In each segment, choose a different aspect of the performance on which to focus, for example, visual, auditory, physical feeling, thoughts, and emotions. Emphasize experiencing that part of your triathlon experience. Then, imagine performing five more times. In these performances, combine all the aspects of imagery and imagine the total performance. The more you can exactly reproduce your actual triathlon experience, the more you'll get from your imagery.

> *Not only should you visualize yourself performing strongly in a perfect race, but you should also visualize things that might go wrong and how you'll deal with them.*
>
> —Wes Hobson, triathlon coach

Imagery for Prime Training

There are several places you can incorporate imagery into your training. Just before you begin a swim set, bike hill repeat, or track interval, instead of thinking about what you want to work on, see and feel yourself doing it with imagery. Close your eyes and briefly imagine how you want to perform. These images will increase your motivation and confidence, raise your intensity, and generate positive thoughts and emotions that will raise the level of your training efforts.

You can also use imagery when you've finished a training segment. If your just-completed training effort was positive, you want to remember the image and feeling. So when you've finished, close your eyes and replay your performance, using imagery to ingrain the positive image and feeling. If your recent effort was poor, the dominant feeling and image is negative. The last thing you want to do is remember it. Yet, that is the image and feeling in your mind and body, and it is what will come out when you begin your next training segment. To flush out the negative image and feeling, right after your last effort, edit your imagery, this time performing well. This editing process clears out the negative image and feeling and replaces it with a positive one.

You can also use imagery after your coach has given you instruction. This type of imagery is most common in swimming, which is the most technical of the three triathlon disciplines and the only one in which most triathletes receive ongoing technical instruction. Typically, a coach will give you feedback and then will tell you to think about it before you begin the next set. But where does thinking occur? In your head. Where does performing occur? In your body. Thinking about instruction doesn't always translate into the body effectively. Imagery acts as a bridge between the thoughts in your mind and the actions in your body. Use imagery to ingrain the instruction into your mind and body. After your coach gives you instruction, close your eyes and imagine yourself making the correction.

I rehearse every scenario of every race in my mind, minute by minute. Before the [2004] Olympic trials I rehearsed the entire race in my mind fifty times—what I wanted to happen, how it would look. The race [trials] happened exactly as I had rehearsed and I got my Olympic berth. It really works for me.

—Victor Plata

DEVELOPING AN IMAGERY PROGRAM

Like any form of training, imagery only has value if used in a consistent and organized way. An imagery program allows you to systematically address key areas you need to improve in each aspect of triathlon. You can use imagery to consistently develop technical, tactical, and mental aspects of your triathlon performance.

Imagery Goals

The first step in developing an imagery program is to set goals. They could be technical, (e.g., improving your swim stroke), tactical (e.g., staying within your prescribed heart rate range), mental (e.g., increasing your confidence), or relate to overall performance (e.g., improving your consistency). Use the Imagery Goals form on page 182 to identify the areas on which you wish to work.

IMAGERY GOALS FORM

Directions: In the space below, indicate your goals for the imagery program. Be specific in identifying areas where you want to improve your triathlon performance.

TECHNICAL

1.

2.

TACTICAL

1.

2.

MENTAL

1.

2.

OVERALL PERFORMANCE

1.

2.

Imagery Ladder

The next step involves creating an imagery performance ladder. Start off doing imagery of training situations where your performance is less important. Using the Imagery Ladder form on page 184, create a ladder of training and race situations in which you'll be performing. The ladder should begin with the least important training situation, for example, a low-key swim workout, and increase up to the most important race that you will compete in during the season. This ladder enables you to work on areas you've identified in increasingly demanding training and race situations.

Begin your imagery program at the lowest rung of the ladder and work your way up until you've reached the highest rung. Don't move up to the next rung until you can perform the way you want at the current rung. Once you feel solid at a particular rung, stay there for several imagery sessions to reinforce the positive images, thoughts, and emotions.

Create Imagery Scenarios

Once you've established your goals and built your imagery ladder, you're ready to create training and race scenarios that you will follow in imagery sessions (see Imagery Scenarios on page 185). These scenarios are actual training and race situations in which you can work on your technical, tactical, mental, and performance goals.

Because triathlon is a sport that requires hours to complete, it would be unrealistic for you to imagine an entire workout or race. Instead, identify four or five specific training or race situations that are realistic that you can imagine for a few minutes each. For example, imagine yourself working on your swim technique while doing a 5 x 50 set, or imagine yourself staying positive and motivated in "snapshots" during the last few miles of the run. As you move up the

I spend the last two weeks before an Ironman working almost exclusively on mental visualization and reinforcing strong mental images of myself. I spend a lot of time visualizing myself as unstoppable, competent, and able to deal with anything thrown my way. I go over, when I am racing, what is important to me about the race. I try and stay away from images such as winning and focus more on being strong throughout, being really tough when things go wrong or get physically uncomfortable.

—Jamie Cleveland,
2000 Ironman® Florida champion

IMAGERY LADDER

Directions: In the space below, create a ladder of training and race situations in which you will imagine yourself. The ladder should increase incrementally in terms of importance. Specify the performance situation (e.g., unstructured workout, focused training session, or race). Examples are italicized.

LEAST IMPORTANT

1. (*training ride with a friend*)

2. (*swim workout with coach*)

MODERATELY IMPORTANT

3. (*training brick as race approaches*)

4. (*low-level race*)

MOST IMPORTANT

5. (*major race*)

IMAGERY SCENARIOS

Directions: In the space below, create several training and race scenarios that you can follow in imagery sessions as you climb the imagery ladder. These scenarios should provide you with detailed descriptions of what you want to imagine as you work on some part of triathlon in training and races.

TRAINING

RACE

imagery ladder, imagine using your improved swim technique or self-talk in increasingly important training and race situations until you can imagine your best performance in the most important race of your season.

Your imagery scenarios should be training and race specific. You shouldn't just imagine yourself performing in a nonspecific location or event, or under undefined conditions. Rather, imagine training and race scenarios in which you perform at a particular site (e.g., a local open-water swim venue), in a specific event (e.g., a triathlon in which you've competed before), under certain conditions (e.g., rough water or a head-wind). Also, be sure that the locations, events, and conditions are appropriate to your level of ability. For example, if you're a middle-of-the-pack age grouper, you shouldn't imagine yourself competing at the ITU World Championships against Craig Walton or Joanna Zeiger.

Imagery Log

Because imagery isn't tangible like weight lifting, where you can see how much weight you've lifted, or speed work, where you can be timed, it's useful to keep a log of your imagery sessions. By recording your imagery sessions, you'll be able to see improvement as you make your way up the ladder. Use the Imagery Log on page 188 to record relevant aspects of your imagery sessions.

The first piece of information to record is the *rung* of your imagery ladder. Place a number between 1 and 5 to indicate where you are in your climb up the ladder. Rate the *quality* of the imagery session on a 1–10 scale. How clear were the images, how well did you perform, how did you feel about the imagery session?

Describe your *performance*, that is, what you worked on and what you actually imagined during the imagery session. Specify the *control* you had in the imagery session. Were your imagined performances of poor or high quality?

Rate the quality of your *senses* in the imagery session. Assign yourself a 1–10 score for how clearly you experienced the visual, auditory, and physical imagery. Finally, evaluate the *mental* aspects of your imagery by briefly describing relevant thoughts and emotions you experienced during your imagery session. The emphasis of this area should be on how positive or negative your thoughts and emotions were during the session.

Practical Concerns

Structure your imagery sessions into your daily routine. If you schedule them for the same time every day, you're more likely to remember to do them. Find a quiet, comfortable place where you won't be disturbed. Each session should last no longer than ten minutes. Do imagery three to four times a week. Like any form of training, if you do it too much, you'll get tired of it. Finally, start your imagery sessions with one of the relaxation procedures that we describe in Chapter 5. The deep state of relaxation will help you generate better-quality images, and it will make you more receptive to the images and feelings you're trying to ingrain.

A few days before the race, I will visualize the race in my head from the very start to finish, including all details like transitions and so on. This allows me to get all of these details into my head. I feel like then I can just go ahead and relax and get rested for the race without constantly thinking about the race.

—Heather Fuhr

IMAGERY LOG

DATE	LADDER # of rung	QUALITY 1–10	PERFORMANCE What you imagined	CONTROL Quality of performance	SENSES Visual—auditory—physical	MENTAL Thoughts and emotions

TRIATHLETE SPOTLIGHT: MARCIA

Marcia considered herself an oddity in the triathlon world. At 62, she was an old lady compared to "youngsters" that populate most races. But she didn't feel old, and her competitive fires still burned brightly. She loved to go against the other "mature" triathletes, and there were several she raced against in the big races with whom she had a heated, though friendly, competition.

Marcia was always looking for ways to get an edge over her competition and, realizing that her body had its limits, she liked to explore how to strengthen her mind. Two years earlier, she had a real scare, having been diagnosed with breast cancer. Fortunately, the cancer was caught early, and after a round of chemotherapy during which she proudly tells people that she didn't miss a day of training, she was pronounced in remission and told to continue her life as before.

During her chemo, Marcia was introduced to healing imagery, a tool she had found helpful during cancer treatment. She used it committedly and believes that it's partly responsible for her return to health. After she got back fully to her tri-life, she decided that if imagery could work with cancer treatment, it could work for triathlon.

Marcia bought a sport psychology book that had a chapter on mental imagery and, following its suggestions, created an imagery program. The two areas she wanted to work on were intensity and pain. Because she was very competitive, she would sometimes get too nervous before races. She also knew that if she wanted to go faster in races, she would have to learn how to deal with pain better.

Marcia scheduled her imagery sessions for Monday, Wednesday, and Friday at 6:15 P.M., just before dinner. In each session, she would start with a relaxation procedure described in the book. To reduce her intensity, she would imagine herself arriving at T1 and going through her pre-race preparations before the race. She would imagine herself feeling confident and using relaxation techniques, such as deep breathing, and calming self-talk, to lower her intensity. To manage her pain better, she would imagine difficult parts of a bike leg and the end of a run leg, pushing herself, being in pain, and using pain-control techniques, such as positive self-talk.

In her first race since starting the imagery program two months earlier, Marcia noticed that she was automatically doing the relaxation

(continued on next page)

(continued from previous page)
strategies she had used in her imagery and felt more relaxed before her start. Late in the race when she was pushing toward the finish, she again found herself using the pain-management techniques naturally and seemed to be able to tolerate more pain as she raced to the finish ahead of her age-group competitors.

PART FOUR

Special Concerns in Triathlon

13 Psychology of Injury

An unfortunate result of the frequency, volume, and intensity of triathlon training is the almost certainty of sustaining an injury at some point during your triathlon participation. Injuries can range from irritating (e.g., a hamstring pull) to frustrating (e.g., plantar fasciitus) to season ending (e.g., torn rotator cuff). They can occur as a result of strength or flexibility imbalances; overuse; poor technique; skeletal misalignment; improper, poorly prepared, or worn equipment; or accidents (e.g., a bike crash or a running fall). The best way to reduce the chances of injuries is with properly fitted and functional equipment; a well-designed conditioning program that combines training for endurance, strength, flexibility, and recovery; sound technical instruction and practice; preventive therapeutic practice (e.g., yoga, stretching, and massage); and discretion while swimming, biking, and running.

Despite your best efforts to prevent injuries, they are almost inevitable. Thankfully, the surgical and rehabilitative technologies have evolved so far in recent years that minor injuries, for example, muscle pulls and tendinitis, can be treated successfully in a short time, and athletes with serious injuries, such as torn ligaments and broken bones, can, in most cases, expect a full recovery and return to sport. However, returning to or surpassing your previous level of performance is not always assured.

Because injuries are fundamentally physical, the focus on recovery is on the repair of the damaged area. Though rehabilitation professionals and athletes alike attest to the mental challenges of an injury, little attention is paid to healing the "mental muscles" that are damaged from the physical injury. Recovery from the mental and emotional harm that was done is what will ultimately enable you to return at a level of performance equal to or above where you were before your injury.

You have several responsibilities in recovering from an injury. Strictly adhere to your physical therapy program. Minimize the deterioration of your preinjury level of fitness. Remain patient so that you give your injury time to heal. Maintain and rehabilitate your mental muscles, including confidence, intensity, focus, and emotions, so that when you return to training, you'll be able to pick up where you left off both physically and mentally.

MOTIVATION

Motivation is the mental factor that influences rehabilitation most directly. Your motivation to follow your physical therapy program will determine its effectiveness. It involves being able to fully adhere to your physical therapy regimen in the face of pain, fatigue, boredom, frustration, impatience, and setbacks. A decline in your motivation will result in a commensurate drop in adherence, which will, in turn, slow your recovery and hinder your return to triathlon. An increase in your motivation may cause you to attempt to accelerate your recovery, overdo your physical therapy, and aggravate the injury.

I think the toughest part [in dealing with injuries] is telling yourself you will get better faster if you rest! Athletes don't like downtime, as they feel their competition is out there making great gains if they are not out training.

—Pete Kain

The motivational strategies described in Chapter 3 that are designed to inspire you in your training can also ensure that you maintain appropriate motivation in your rehabilitation. Setting goals, having variety in your physical therapy program, continuing your conditioning program, focusing on a complete return to triathlon, and receiving support from others can help you maintain your motivation when you get discouraged. The same attitude and approach that keeps you from overtraining can also prevent you from trying to speed up your recovery. Understanding that healing takes time, trusting your rehab program, maintaining balance in your life by doing other things while injured, keeping perspective on how triathlon fits into your life, and avoiding overinvestment can ensure that you maintain a healthy level of motivation.

CONFIDENCE

How strongly you believe that you can recover and return to triathlon may be the single most important mental contributor to a full recovery. Lack of confidence can plunge you into a deep pit of despair that slows your rehabilitation and makes your recovery painful physically and mentally. High confidence can propel you into an upward spiral of hope, determination, and positive thinking.

Types of confidence. There are several areas in which you need to have confidence to maximize its benefits in your rehabilitation. As you begin your rehabilitation, have confidence in your physical therapy program. A simple question to ask yourself is, "Do I believe this regimen will enable me to recover fully and as quickly as possible?" If you can't answer in the affirmative, you should speak to your sports medicine professional to be convinced of the program's effectiveness, or find another expert you can trust.

You also need to reinstill physical confidence in the injured area. Once you sustain an injury, you may question whether the damaged area can withstand the demands of performance when you return to triathlon. Though your physical confidence is challenged and bolstered every day when you're healthy, an injury communicates to you that your body may no longer be capable of meeting that challenge. Rehabilitation should be a daily reaffirmation of your physical confidence in which you're proving to yourself once again that your body will sustain itself under the physical stress of triathlon. As healing occurs and function returns, physical confidence must incrementally improve until you have a complete belief in your body's ability to return to its previous level of performance. Staying as active as possible during rehabilitation and acknowledging progress as you heal are two ways to foster physical confidence.

Your final mental hurdle is regaining your confidence that you can perform at or above the level you were prior to the injury. Return-to-triathlon confidence is your belief that the formerly injured area is now fully rehabilitated and healed, you're physically and mentally prepared for the rigors of training, and you can return to a high level of competitive performance. Return-to-triathlon confidence evolves from sustained program and physical confidence, a positive and successful rehabilitation program, maintaining your fitness and technical skills during recovery, and using mental training techniques to keep your mind sharp and focused. A progression of rehabilitation and return-to-triathlon imagery that is consistent and builds on daily progress will also increase confidence steadily with few declines.

Rehabilitating the confidence muscle. Confidence can be thought of as a muscle that, like the physically injured area, also becomes injured. If your confidence muscle isn't rehabilitated along with the damaged area, your ability to return fully to training and racing will be compromised. An injured confidence muscle expresses itself as negative thinking, emotions, and physiology, all of which can act as obstacles to your complete and timely return to triathlon. The injury may cause you to doubt whether your body is capable of handling the demands placed on it. It may also cause you to question whether you will be able to perform at a high level again. The injured confidence muscle can produce a negative attitude toward rehabilitation and your return to the sport. Engaging in confidence-building "therapy" will ensure that your confidence muscle heals and is well conditioned when you return to triathlon training and racing.

A lot of people had written me off [due to injury] and it got under my skin. But I maintained a big belief in myself. I knew I was still dangerous.
—Loretta Harrop,
2004 Olympics silver medalist

The confidence-building strategies discussed in Chapter 4 that are designed to improve your triathlon performance can also be used to rehabilitate your confidence muscle. Viewing your injury as a form of adversity, receiving support from family, friends, and training buddies, and acknowledging small successes in physical therapy act as a foundation for maintaining your confidence during rehabilitation. You can then use specific techniques that guard against discouragement and bolster your confidence, such as positive self-talk and body language, confidence keywords, optimistic thinking, and mental imagery in which you see and feel yourself healing and getting stronger.

STRESS

The stress you experience from being injured and not being able to train and race can interfere with your rehabilitation. You can think of stress as a negative mental and physical response to a perceived threat, in your case, not being able to do something you love. Stress occurs when you view your injury and the subsequent rehabilitation as a threat to your physical health, sense of self-worth, and happiness.

Stress hurts the six mental factors of the Prime Triathlon pyramid. Stress can hurt your confidence and motivation by creating discomfort and doubt about your recovery. It can also direct your focus onto negative aspects of your injury rather than on positive aspects of your recovery. Stress from injury can cause unpleasant emotions, including fear, frustration, and despair. The physical price of injury-related stress can include increased muscle tension and bracing, greater pain, difficulty sleeping, loss of appetite, and slowed healing.

Lowering your stress will allow you to feel more positive, relaxed, and comfortable, and will encourage faster healing and recovery. You can reduce the stress you experience during your rehabilitation by using the psych-down techniques we discuss in Chapter 5, including deep breathing, muscle relaxation, maintaining focus on the healing process, listening to relaxing music, being with supportive people, and participating in other activities that you enjoy.

FOCUS

Focus is an underappreciated, yet essential, mental contributor to rehabilitation. Too often triathletes can spend more time focusing on the injury and what they can't do rather than on the recovery and what they can and will be able to do. Having a negative focus can reduce confidence and motivation, increase stress, and result in a preoccupation with negative emotions, such as fear, frustration, and sadness. A positive and constructive focus fosters an overall mind-set that encourages healing and a timely return to triathlon.

The strategies we discuss in Chapter 6 can be used to enhance focus. Keywords, focusing on things over which you have control, and maintaining a long-term focus on rehabilitation help to create this positive mind-set.

Of particular value are the four P's that we describe in Chapter 6; a focus that emphasizes the positive aspects of rehabilitation, the present, the process, and progress encouragingly affects the other Prime Triathlon pyramid factors, as well as the rehabilitation as a whole.

EMOTIONS

Of all the mental areas that are affected by an injury, emotions may be the most acutely experienced. The shock and pain that accompanies an injury and the anxiety about what it means to your future triathlon participation can create a veritable maelstrom of emotional upset. The emotions you may feel can include irritation, frustration, fear, sadness, devastation, and despair. The intensity of these emotions will depend on how serious the injury is, how invested you are in triathlon, and how much it disrupts your active lifestyle.

For you to have a complete and manageable rehabilitation, you need to minimize these negative emotions and replace them as much as possible with positive emotions. The challenge is that it's difficult to feel positive emotions, such as excitement or joy, about an occurrence that is far from pleasant. For your own emotional well-being, as well as for progress in your rehabilitation, you can, nonetheless, foster hope in your return to health, inspiration to motivate your rehabilitation efforts, and pride in your progress back to triathlon. Realistically, though, feeling such good emotions consistently may be hard to achieve when you're injured, so the best you may be able to hope for is to balance your emotional scales. This involves accepting that you're going to feel unpleasant emotions periodically, particularly when you are tired, in pain, or experiencing a setback. At the same time, look for opportunities in which you can generate positive emotions about your recovery.

In Chapter 7, we discuss at length the role of emotions in triathlon performance and focus on three negative emotions—fear, frustration, and despair—that are most influential in the sport. These same emotions can affect you even more noticeably when you're injured because injury is a significant threat to your physical and mental health and well-being. You can use the perspectives and strategies described in Chapter 7 to help you manage the emotions you feel in response to your injury, rehabilitation, and return to triathlon.

The emotional challenges you face do not end when your physical therapist announces that you're healed and ready to return to triathlon. When you first return to the setting in which you became injured, you may experience fear of reinjury. This reaction is normal given that your last experience wasn't a positive one. Preventing fear of reinjury should be a part of your rehabilitation program and include the mental training strategies that we discuss in the book.

Fear of reinjury is most commonly caused by an incomplete recovery. This problem is exacerbated when you still have physical deficits associated with the injury, for example, reduced strength or limited range of motion. In this case, your concern about reinjury is legitimate and you should speak to your sports medicine professional about whether you are ready to return to triathlon training. Your belief that rehabilitation wasn't effective can be just as difficult. These doubts may be caused by complications or setbacks that slowed your recovery, causing you to question how well you've healed and how prepared you are to return to triathlon. This lack of trust in the injured area will affect you physically (e.g., anxiety and bracing) and mentally (e.g., low motivation, poor confidence, lack of focus, and tentative effort), not only causing a fear of reinjury, but also increasing the chances of reinjury.

Overzealousness in your desire to return to triathlon can also cause a fear of reinjury. If you become impatient and try to rush back to training, you may do too much too soon, placing demands on your body that it is not ready to handle. This eagerness can then result in reinjury or compensatory injury to a related area. Impatience can actually slow your return rather than achieving the intended goal of a faster return to the sport.

You can prevent fear of reinjury by rehabilitating the mental muscles, such as confidence, stress, and focus, with the strategies we discuss in this chapter, maintaining a rigorous conditioning program around the injury and using mental imagery during rehabilitation (these topics will be discussed in greater depth shortly). Perhaps the most important way to prevent fear of reinjury is a timely, disciplined, and steady return to triathlon when your physical therapist fully clears you to resume training. This progressive approach enables you to slowly expose the rehabilitated area, and your mind and body in general, to incrementally greater demands in training. With successful early experiences in your return to triathlon, you can regain your trust that you are once again ready for high-level training and competition.

Though some fear of reinjury is normal and may pass as you reacquaint yourself with training, we recommend a proactive approach so fear doesn't interfere with a timely and complete return. A fear reaction is common when you first put yourself in the situation in which you were injured. You can reduce your initial fear by reentering the situation gradually, for example, testing the formerly injured area at lower volume and intensity and building up as you regain trust and comfort. Each successful experience in this progression reduces your fear of reinjury and reaffirms to you that the healed area is once again capable of sustaining itself under the demands of performance.

Discussing your fears with your physician or physical therapist and other triathletes who have returned from similar injuries can also allay your apprehension and help you gain a positive, realistic, and healthy perspective as you return to training. These conversations can be beneficial by showing you that what you're thinking and feeling are normal and expected parts of rehabilitation. You may also learn useful strategies to help you through the transition. These discussions can also remind you of why you worked so hard to rehabilitate, the importance of a complete return to health and participation in triathlon, and your commitment to renewing training and surpassing your previous level of performance.

PAIN

All triathletes are accustomed to the discomfort of training and racing. Anyone who pushes him or herself has learned to deal with the pain experienced from such efforts. But pain from injury is an added dimension to the physical challenges you face in triathlon. As we discussed in Chapter 8, injury pain differs from exertion pain in that it is usually more severe, not readily controllable, and continues after you've halted your efforts.

Injury pain plays an important role in your rehabilitation and return to triathlon by affecting the other Prime Triathlon pyramid factors. Uncontrolled pain can hamper your motivation and reduce your physical therapy efforts. It can be discouraging and hurt your confidence. Pain is a powerful pull on your focus and can foster unpleasant emotions about your recovery. Injury pain affects you physically by creating muscle tension, restricting oxygen intake and blood flow, and slowing healing. Managing your pain will allow you to feel less pain and encourage a bodily state that is more receptive to rehabilitation and healing. Pain management will also give you a greater sense of control, reduce stress, and increase motivation, confidence, and focus.

The same strategies that were discussed in Chapter 8 to manage training and race pain can be used successfully in dealing with injury pain. Having a realistic perspective, understanding, and interpretation of pain can change your attitude toward injury pain. Using pain as useful information and generating positive self-talk and emotions can take the edge off of the pain by inducing a more relaxed state, which can actually reduce the pain you experience during your rehabilitation.

FACILITATING REHABILITATION

In addition to the many techniques that we just described that you can use to bolster the Prime Triathlon pyramid, there are several other strategies that can support your rehabilitation and facilitate your return to triathlon. Consistent with our discussion of injury so far, some of these approaches are addressed in more detail in other parts of the book.

Rehabilitation as Athletic Performance

You can bolster your recovery by recognizing that "rehabilitation is athletic performance" and that you already possess many of the skills to successfully complete rehabilitation. The same qualities that enable you to pursue your triathlon goals, namely, the six factors in the Prime Triathlon pyramid (motivation, confidence, intensity, focus, emotions, and pain), can be used to enhance your recovery from injury. Also, all of the information and strategies that we discuss in this book about enhancing triathlon performance can be used to facilitate recovery from injury. If you apply the same kind of commitment, diligence, and energy that you put toward triathlon and use the many mental training techniques we describe in this book, you will be back in the pool, on the bike, and in your running shoes before you know it.

Train around Your Injury

One of the fears that triathletes have when they take time off to recover from an injury is that they will lose the fitness that they worked so long and hard to achieve. A powerful way you can keep yourself positive mentally and sharp physically is to train around your injury. This means that you should continue to improve your fitness in ways that don't aggravate your injury, for example, kicking in the pool while allowing shoulder tendinitis to heal or doing water running while suffering from shin splints.

Continuing your conditioning program has both physical and mental benefits. We've known triathletes who have come back to the sport in better physical condition than prior to their injury because they focused on aspects of their training that they had previously neglected. You can also reduce the frustration you might feel that you're losing your fitness and no longer pursuing your triathlon goals by continuing to train around your injury. Engaging in a vigorous conditioning program will foster your motivation to rehab, build your confidence for when you return to the sport, reduce your anxiety about being injured, help you focus on healing rather than being injured, and generate feelings of hope and inspiration from your efforts.

Patience

Perhaps your greatest challenge in rehabilitation is staying patient and not trying to rush back to training and racing. Losing patience is particularly noticeable for minor injuries, such as muscle pulls and tendinitis, which hurt, but don't necessarily prevent you from training. Realize that it is difficult to work through an injury. Injuries rarely heal themselves, particularly if you continue to do what caused the injury in the first place.

I have learned the hard way that trying to train through an injury will only prolong it, as well as usually create a secondary injury. So using my own experience has made me better at telling myself to back off and rest.

—Pete Kain

If you're like most triathletes, you may try to ignore the injury or hope that it goes away. But if the injury persists and causes considerable pain, you'll have to get over your denial and accept that you're injured. The first step is to take a few days off and do RICE (rest, ice, compression, elevation). During these initial days, you may feel frustrated and antsy, and feel compelled to train again even though you know you shouldn't. If you have these urges, remind yourself that a few days of rest now is better than a few weeks off later because you didn't allow the injury to heal. Enlisting family and friends to talk sense into you can also help.

If the injury doesn't heal after a few days, it's time to see a sports medicine professional who can properly diagnose and treat the injury. In a way, a minor injury is harder to deal with than a severe injury because with the latter you have no choice but to stop training. But with a minor injury you can delude yourself and continue to train even if it will only aggravate the injury. Patience is again the key. The marvelous thing about physical therapy is that, in most cases, if you adhere to the rehab program, you heal. The frustrating thing is that you can't rush recovery; your body needs to be allowed the time to heal.

Rehabilitation Imagery

Mental imagery is a powerful tool for enhancing your recovery. Seeing and feeling yourself rehabilitate and return to triathlon triggers a variety of mental and physical responses that can help you get back to training and racing more quickly and better prepared. Imagery can benefit you mentally by protecting the Prime Triathlon pyramid. There is evidence that imagery can augment physical healing as well. You can use four types of mental imagery to maximize its benefits in your rehabilitation and return to triathlon.

- **Healing imagery** involves imagining the damaged area mending and healing. Gain a clear picture of the injured area and what it looks like when healed. This can be done with the use of illustrations, X-rays, or MRIs of the injured area. Over the period of rehabilitation, healing imagery may physiologically facilitate healing, but just as importantly, it will bolster your confidence and trust that the injured area is healing fully.

- **Soothing imagery** can be useful for lessening pain. You can see and feel yourself in a calm and peaceful place, for example, floating on a cloud or laying on a beach. Soothing imagery reduces sympathetic nervous system activity, muscle tension, and other symptoms of stress that can cause pain. It can take your focus away from the pain and onto more enjoyable images and feelings. The soothing images can foster positive emotions that will also ease the pain.

- **Performance imagery** is important during rehabilitation because it counters the belief you might have that your triathlon development is being interrupted. Performance imagery is a way for you to continue your progress in the areas of technique, tactics, and mental preparation while you're recovering from injury. A program of performance imagery sessions in which you see and feel yourself swimming, biking, and running can help reduce the "mental atrophy" that can occur while you're away from the sport.

• **Return-to-triathlon imagery,** an extension of performance imagery, is most useful as you approach the conclusion of your rehabilitation. The value of return-to-triathlon imagery is that it enables you to practice your reintroduction to triathlon training and performance before you actually return to the pool, bike, or track. This imagined rehearsal generates successful images and feelings that enhance familiarity and comfort, increase motivation, bolster confidence, create a constructive focus, reduce anxiety, and foster positive emotions associated with your return. Adding relaxation techniques (described in Chapter 5) before beginning return-to-triathlon imagery can further facilitate this process by inducing a positive physical state to accompany the positive images, thoughts, and emotions. You can use the information and tools in Chapter 9 to implement a mental imagery program that incorporates healing, soothing, performance, and return-to-triathlon imagery.

Social Support

When you get injured, you often remove yourself from an environment that is reinforcing (e.g., masters swims, group rides, track workouts) at a time when you most need support. Social support can offer you a meaningful connection with those who care about you that fosters positive emotions, provides encouragement during difficult times, and promotes sharing with others. It ensures that you have access to relevant information about your rehabilitation. Social support gives you the feeling that you have people to help you get through a difficult time.

Your three primary sources of support are your sports medicine team, members of your training circle, and family and friends. Each of these groups can offer you different, yet equally important, types of support. The sports medicine team can give you technical support directly related to your rehabilitation that can facilitate your recovery. Your training circle can encourage and motivate you to continue your efforts and offer shared emotional support. Family and friends can also give you emotional support and enable you to openly express concerns and feelings you may not feel comfortable sharing with others. All three groups can help you maintain a positive attitude and foster more positive emotions, such as caring, hope, and humor. When you're injured, there can be a tendency to want to withdraw from people, but we encourage you to actively seek out support from those around you.

Remarkable Recovery

A compelling aspect of injury rehabilitation is termed "remarkable recovery," which is distinguished by the speed of rehabilitation, decisive conquest over physical challenges, and a return to sport at a level higher than prior to the injury. The quality of recovery from an injury depends on a number of physical aspects of the injury, including severity, preinjury physical fitness, individual healing ability, and effectiveness of the rehabilitation program. Research has also suggested that certain mental factors can contribute to the speed and quality of recovery.

Research found that injured athletes who had unusually fast recoveries used positive self-talk, goal setting, social support, and healing imagery significantly more than athletes who had slow or average recoveries. There was also some evidence to suggest that athletes who recovered more quickly were more optimistic, had a more positive attitude, and experienced less stress than those who recovered more slowly. Athletes who had remarkable recoveries also had greater personal control and responsibility for their injuries and used more mental strategies to bolster their recoveries. The exceptional healers were also less fearful of reinjury, and when they did feel some fear, they actively took steps to allay their concerns. Finally, athletes who recovered more quickly expressed that the injury and rehabilitation were valuable learning experiences that enhanced their enjoyment and performance when they returned to their sport. The value of these attributes associated with remarkable recovery is that they're within your control and you can readily use them in your rehabilitation.

TRIATHLETE SPOTLIGHT: CARL

Carl, a 36-year-old, was seen by all who knew him as a person who was maniacally committed to triathlon. For the past eight years, he had trained with focused zeal and raced as often as he could. Neither work nor weather nor illness could keep him from his workouts.

A week before an upcoming Olympic-distance race, Carl turned his ankle while on a trail run. He still completed the run, but limped home in considerable pain. Assuming it was nothing serious, he thought that he could work through it and be ready for the race. The next day it was swollen and hurt a lot, but he still went to his masters swim and spinning

(continued on next page)

(continued from previous page)

class. His ankle hurt like hell, but he didn't think he could hurt it more. The next day, he jogged in pain through a 3-mile run. Three days before the race, he still walked with a limp, but, being a "hard" guy, figured he could tough it out.

The race, not surprisingly, didn't go well. Carl got through the swim okay, though his kick was nonexistent. He had to back off his bike because pushing hard on his pedals caused his ankle to hurt a lot. And the run was a total failure; he was in such pain that he walked the first mile and had to abandon the race before mile 2. He went home dejected at DNFing for the first time in his triathlon life.

Carl finally got the message that his ankle was hurt worse than he was willing to admit. The next day he visited a physical therapist and was diagnosed with a second-degree sprain. The PT, Emily, prescribed five days on crutches, daily physical therapy, RICE, anti-inflammatories, and no running or biking for at least two weeks. Emily also warned Carl that he should expect to not be at full strength for at least a month. He was crushed at hearing that he couldn't train as usual and had to drop out of an upcoming race.

Emily told Carl that how quickly he recovered depended on his commitment to the physical therapy regimen and his attitude toward his recovery. Emily suggested that he think of rehab as just like training and recommended a program that would help him get back out there as soon as possible.

In addition to the rehab plan, Emily created a physical training program that he could do to help maintain his fitness. It included masters swims with a buoy in which he didn't kick, water running, and water "cycling," which simulated the pedaling motion. Carl also continued his weight lifting, doing his usual workout minus any weight-bearing exercises, such as leg presses. He also decided to take a few swim lessons to improve his technique, something he'd wanted to do for a long time but could never find the time. Staying so active and actually improving himself enabled him to feel less stressed about his time away from triathlon and to maintain a better attitude than he expected.

Emily also gave Carl several articles about the mental side of injury rehab and suggested that he do some of the exercises they described. One recommendation that he took to was to imagine himself performing in different parts of a race. The images of swimming, biking, and running really psyched him up and helped him stay positive. His biggest challenge was his impatience, but to counteract his urge to rush his rehab, he followed one of the article's recommendations by writing notes to himself with messages saying "patience," "give it time," and "healing can't be rushed."

Wanting to stay involved, Carl volunteered to organize an aid station for a nearby triathlon. Though it was difficult for him to be on the sidelines, he enjoyed supporting the competitors that day and it gave him a new perspective on what it's like to race a triathlon. Whenever he talked about going for "just a short run," his training buddy, Dave, would slap him upside his head (literally) and tell him, "Don't even think about it."

Though the weeks went by slowly, his ankle was improving; the swelling went down and the pain had subsided somewhat. Carl also found that he was enjoying the new physical conditioning program he was on. The imagery was helping his attitude, and he found himself less antsy about getting back to training.

After three weeks, Emily told Carl it was time to get back to biking and running, albeit slowly and only for short distances. Having seen vast improvement in his ankle so far, he wasn't about to screw it up again, so he followed Emily's plan to the letter. Each week, his ankle felt better and better; the swelling was gone, there was almost no pain, and it felt stable again.

Finally, after six weeks, Emily set Carl free; he could get back to training at his usual crazy intensity, except no trail running for two more months. Much to his surprise, he felt strong from his first day back. In his first race, a month later, his ankle felt great and he had a better result than expected. He actually felt like he was stronger than before he hurt his ankle. He sent Emily a heartfelt thank-you card and sang praises about her to all of his friends.

14 Ironman Preparation and Racing

Ironman is the ultimate in triathlon competition. It's the standard by which triathlon is known to the world at large. Almost every non-tri person you meet will ask you whether you've done an Ironman (that's all they know), as if that is the only badge of honor in triathlon. Within our sport, Ironman competitors are accorded a certain reverence. Because of its status as the greatest challenge in the sport, the pull of doing an Ironman can be strong if you take your participation seriously or want the recognition and validation that being an Ironman finisher accords. Putting in the training time, going the distance, crossing the line as an Ironman finisher (even qualifying for Kona!) are all heady stuff that can act as a siren's call to triathletes.

But should you do an Ironman? Training for and finishing an Ironman can be a uniquely positive, life-enriching experience that fosters passion, physical health, and deep friendships. It can also be a source of personal, work, and social stress, a cause of injuries, and a less than satisfying experience in which the costs outweigh the benefits. Which experience you have will depend on why you want to do an Ironman, how it will affect your life, and what you expect to get out of it. We encourage you to give careful thought to this question to make sure that if you choose to do an Ironman, you do it for reasons that are healthy and beneficial. The following is some food for thought in making your decision about whether to enter an Ironman.

"WRONG" REASONS

Despite its positive atmosphere, Ironman can be an obsessive, narcissistic, and self-indulgent pursuit. Because of the time and energy that's required, it can cause you to sacrifice work, alienate family and friends, narrow your life, and harm you physically. As noble a quest as Ironman can be, it can be an unhealthy, corrupting influence if viewed through an overly myopic and self-absorbed lens.

We live in a "more is better" culture. You can fall into the trap of "If I feel good doing an Olympic, I'll feel even better doing a half-Ironman, and if I feel that good doing a half, I'll feel even better doing an Ironman." But we often forget that, like most things, triathlon can have a point of diminishing returns; longer distances won't necessarily give you greater benefits in terms of enjoyment, fitness, or fulfillment. Is Ironman even enough? There is XTERRA, double-Ironman races, ultramarathoning, Eco-Challenge, and Mount Everest! There is always a greater challenge, but is it healthy to always be setting the bar higher?

We also live in a culture in which many people are looking for that elusive something called happiness. They engage in activities to fill a void left by unsatisfying work and bad relationships. People do things that they hope will build their self-esteem, relieve their loneliness, ease their anxiety, and make them feel good about themselves. Triathlon can be one of those activities. These people immerse themselves in the sport hoping to find answers to questions that they have been asking for many years. When they don't find it at the Olympic distance, they may assume that they just aren't going far enough. When the answers continue to elude them, they believe that the answers can only be found in an Ironman. But if you're looking for answers to your life's questions in Ironman, you may end up frustrated and unsatisfied because, though it can offer meaning, satisfaction, and joy, the answers to life will, in all likelihood, not be found in an Ironman.

In addition to our eternal search for happiness, many people are also looking for respect and acceptance from others. As one Ironman triathlete put it, "I wanted to tell people that I did one," in the belief that others would hold him in greater esteem and that he would be more popular, particularly, as he noted, with women. Though there are people who treat others better because of their accomplishments, saying that you have done an Ironman is unlikely to produce deeper and more meaningful relationships. The time, energy, and discomfort of training for and competing in an Ironman are also probably not worth the fleeting perception that you're extra special for having done one.

"RIGHT" REASONS

There are many good reasons for doing an Ironman. Ironman is about facing and overcoming physical and mental challenges you may not otherwise have the opportunity to face in your life. It involves extending yourself beyond what you thought was possible and finding physical and mental strengths that you may not have known existed. The experiences you have in your Ironman pursuits can free you from formerly self-imposed limitations in other areas of your life. It can change the way you look at yourself, causing you to throw off old, potentially unhealthy beliefs about yourself. Ironman can inspire you, give you confidence, improve your focus, show you how to manage your emotions better, and help you learn to overcome pain. Ironman can teach you lessons about patience, perseverance, persistence, adversity, and flexibility that can benefit you in your work, relationships, and other activities. You can get great joy out of your Ironman experience, and it can enrich an already good life. Ironman can give your life new meaning, depth, and connectedness.

Ironman, if done for the right reasons, can change your relationships and your social world. With almost complete unanimity, professional and age-group triathletes alike emphasize the people they meet when they talk about what they get most out of their Ironman experiences: the camaraderie and the bond that they feel with other Ironman triathletes. Ironman training is very social: masters swims, long rides and runs, and track workouts. Ironman races are noted for their social activities: the pre- and post-race banquets, meals out, the athlete village, the race itself, and the respect shared among athletes taking on the same enormous task. Ironman has the potential to offer you deep and lasting relationships with people who share your values, interests, and goals.

KNOW WHAT YOU'RE GETTING INTO

Choosing to train for an Ironman should be a thoughtful and deliberate choice based on a clear understanding of what's involved, its benefits and costs, and what you will ultimately gain from the experience. Because an Ironman is such a time- and energy-intensive endeavor, it's important to know what you're getting into before you decide to take the plunge. Ironman isn't just a race that occurs on a particular date. Rather, it's a lifestyle that involves many choices that can affect all aspects of your life. The choices that Ironman requires you to make are neither right nor wrong; they are simply ones that must be made if you decide to pursue an Ironman.

In this section, we want to show you the different faces of Ironman, not just the bright and smiling face you most often see. Only you can decide whether an Ironman is right for you. By showing you all sides of Ironman, we want to help you make an informed decision about why you would want to participate and what you expect to gain from the time, energy, and money you devote. After reading this section, we want you to ask yourself two questions. First, do you want to do an Ironman for the right reasons? Second, within your overall life picture, will an Ironman be worth it?

In a decidedly nonscientific survey Jim conducted online with the Golden Gate Triathlon Club (GGTC) in San Francisco in summer 2004, numerous respondents shared their experiences about the costs and benefits of doing an Ironman. The results are shared below to help you make these choices in a well-informed and considered way.

Time

The most notable aspect of committing to an Ironman is that it's time consuming. Expect that, for six months, your life will revolve around Ironman. Weekly training will range from ten to twenty-plus hours. Most days will involve morning and end-of-day workouts of swimming, biking, or running. You also find time for strength training, stretching, and perhaps yoga and massage. If you have a "real" job, as most prospective Ironman triathletes do, you'll be getting up very early and finishing your workouts in the evening. Toward the peak of your training, your weekends will be filled with training. Saturdays will typically be devoted to long rides or a long swim-bike or bike-run brick. These workouts can take up to eight hours to complete. Sundays aren't quite as time consuming, typically three to four hours, and are usually composed of a long run or a swim-run brick.

Energy

Ironman training is physically demanding. At the height of your training you'll be tired most of the time. You'll want to go to bed early, particularly if you have early-morning workouts. Most triathlon coaches recommend naps during the most intense parts of your Ironman training program, though most prospective Ironman athletes don't have time to sleep during the day. You'll be hungry a great deal. The sheer volume of energy you burn requires constant replenishment. Because of the volume and intensity of training, your immune system may be vulnerable and you could get sick more easily and more often, particularly during your longest, most intense training in the few months before your race. Injuries can be a common part of the Ironman lifestyle because of the frequency, volume, and intensity of training, and the excessive demands you place on your body.

Expense

Triathlon in general is an expensive sport and Ironman is even more costly. An understanding of the financial commitment should be a part of your decision making. The entry fee for an Ironman ranges from around $300 for Iron-distance (but not Ironman-brand) races and some international Ironman events to over $400 for North American Ironman-brand races. Though you may race your Ironman on the same bike you've been using for your shorter-distance triathlons, if you're like many prospective Ironman competitors, you may want to upgrade your bike, which can range from $2,000 to $5,000. Necessary swim, bike, and run gear, including tires and tubes, wet suits, swimsuits, goggles, and running shoes, will range from $500 to $3,000. Your monthly food bill will increase dramatically because of the voracious appetite that Ironman training causes. You may also spend a considerable amount of money on nutritional supplements, including energy drinks, bars, and gels, and electrolyte tablets ($200 to $1,000). Many Ironman entrants hire a triathlon coach (either in person or online), which can cost anywhere from $50 to over $500 a month, to provide them with a training program and moral support, as well as take swim lessons, spin classes, and bike and running clinics. Others join triathlon clubs or Ironman training groups, which also have dues or fees ranging from $50 to $100, that offer structured training opportunities. Pool and track privileges range from $100 to $500. You may also want various forms of physiological, nutritional, and biomechanical testing to ensure you're maximizing your training efforts ($100 to $1000). Because injuries can be a common part of Ironman training, you may need to include visits to your sports medicine physician, physical therapist, or massage therapist (depends on insurance; average: $250).

Prospective Ironman competitors typically race in several shorter warm-up triathlons, swim events, century rides, and running races for which you will incur entry fees and travel costs ranging from $100 to $1,500. It is also common for Ironman triathletes to attend training camps ($150 to $1,500). Because of the time you will spend on your bike, a professional bike fit, which can cost from $75 to $400, is a must, plus bike maintenance at around $75 per tune-up in most bike shops. And don't forget the triathlon books, magazines, and videotapes from which you may want to learn more about Ironman ($15 to $100).

You would incur many of these expenses racing only shorter-distance races. However, because Ironman training is a much bigger commitment, triathletes typically put more into it, including higher-quality gear, coaching, camps, and supplements. Ironman also requires four times the mileage of Olympic-distance training, so many of these expenses (e.g., tires and tubes, running shoes, and nutrition) rise over shorter-course racing.

Getting to and staying at Ironman events adds expense as well. Unless you're close enough to drive to the race, you will have to pay for airfare, airline bike fees, or shipping, rental car, lodging, and food (ranging from $200 for a local race to $3,000 for international events). And don't forget all of the Ironman-brand clothing and gear you will certainly buy at the race expo ($75 to $500). Finally, race photos to commemorate your finish are an absolute must once you get home ($25 to $150). If you get hooked, you'd better include these expenses in your budgeting for years to come.

Several respondents gave detailed accountings of their Ironman expenses. Not including a new bike, yearly costs ranged from about $1,000 for a local, Iron-distance race to over $12,000 for an international Ironman-brand event, with an average of $6,400. Finally, as one GGTC Ironman triathlete put it, "Swim—$600, bike—$2,700, run—$300, travel—$1,000, intense suffering for 10 to 17 hours—priceless!"

These expenses will be offset somewhat by money you would ordinarily spend in other areas during your Ironman training; during periods of high-volume training, you'll be spending most of your time sleeping, eating, training, and working. You may save money by not going to restaurants, movies, bars, or on vacations (though vacations are often combined with an Ironman). As the GGTC survey suggested, you may also save money on dating because you won't have the time or energy to date, and few people will want to date someone who spends so much time training.

Opportunity Costs

In the survey, the most common response about the costs of an Ironman surprisingly didn't have to do with out-of-pocket expenses. Instead, most of the respondents mentioned the opportunity costs of doing an Ironman. Opportunity costs is an economics term that involves *the cost of something in terms of an opportunity foregone.* For example, if you decide to do an Ironman, the opportunity cost is what you might otherwise do with the time, energy, and money you commit to it. The respondents expressed two opportunity costs that were most significant to them: work and relationships.

Because of the time commitment that an Ironman requires, you may have to make sacrifices somewhere. You may not work as long or as hard as usual. If you work for others, you're likely to arrive late, take long lunches, and leave early. Because you'll often be tired, hungry, or simply distracted by Ironman, your productivity may decline. If you work for yourself, you can expect to make less money in your Ironman year because the time you spend training and traveling will be time away from earning a living.

The most frequently raised issue from the GGTC survey was the sacrifices that Ironman triathletes made in their relationships. Your relationships with family and friends will be tested because you will have to choose your training over social activities. You may alienate loved ones and lose touch with friends who are not involved in the sport. Several respondents, when they added up the total financial costs of their Ironman, gave the dollar amount and then added "plus one girlfriend," who they lost because of their commitment to Ironman. Others indicated how pursuing an Ironman put strain on their marriages and families. The time that you spend training is time away from spouses, children, and friends. Some of the respondents said that they had become expert negotiators, trading training time in exchange for chores around the house. To be fair, several respondents indicated how much support they received from their families and friends, and Jim met his wife, who is also a triathlete, while preparing for his first Ironman. They feel positive about exposing their children to the healthy attitudes and lifestyle of Ironman life.

Stress and Emotions

Ironman is psychologically and emotionally taxing and can be stressful. In addition to the stress from the time and energy devoted to the training itself, Ironman can create stress at work and in your relationships from time pressures, required sacrifices, and energy deficits. Additionally, due to the ongoing and intense physical strain you place on your body, you may experience fatigue, exhaustion, overtraining, or burnout, which can cause you to be more emotionally sensitive and to feel irritable and depressed more than usual.

Benefits

Our intention is to offer you a realistic depiction of the costs and benefits of an Ironman. Clearly, there is a tremendous upside for triathletes, as they enter Ironman races in record numbers (races usually fill up within weeks of the opening of registration). The respondents to the GGTC survey offered some largely intangible, though no less compelling, examples of what they got out of their Ironman experiences.

To preface, we try to present "ups" that are not apparent or as strong in shorter-course training and races. You don't need to be an Ironman to gain the benefits of fitness, being outdoors, making friends, traveling, or pushing yourself to greater heights. The themes we discuss below are most relevant and powerful for Ironman triathletes.

The most notable "up" that we hear from Ironman finishers is the relationships that are built in training and the race. As one GGTC member put it, those who pursue an Ironman "belong to a kind of family. We understand the shared support that's needed, the shared insecurities that arise, the shared sense of accomplishment, the shared pain of disappointment. I've never witnessed as much empathy, generosity, and genuine concern among strangers than I did on race day." The long hours of training and the shared ongoing and intense exertion that Ironman triathletes put forth cement a bond that simply doesn't exist in shorter-distance races.

Another meaningful theme that we have seen is the wish for Ironman triathletes to present themselves with a monumental challenge to face and overcome. Many triathletes who enter an Ironman see it as an impossible dream. Yet they choose to chase that dream despite its immense difficulty. Only after many months of training does the initial impossibility become a possibility. The experience of training for and finishing an Ironman shows them that the limits they—and others—place on themselves are more perception than reality. This process of broadening what is seen as possible carries over into all aspects of their lives. Said one GGTC Ironman triathlete, expressing one reason why she does them, "To say 'up yours' to people who said I couldn't do it!"

One triathlete observed that Ironman competitors don't let life just go by. They push beyond their comfort zones. A quote from author Jack London expresses the Ironman perspective well, "It's so much easier to live a quiet and comfortable life. But to live a quiet and comfortable life is not to live at all." Ironman triathletes thrive on the uncomfortable and enjoy exploring unknown territory physically and psychologically. This "stretching" expands the range of experiences to which they are willing to expose themselves and opens up a much larger and richer world in which to live. They feel most alive, vital, and connected to life when they're challenging themselves and striving to reach new heights.

Another theme that has emerged is the importance of goals in the lives of Ironman competitors. Another GGTC member says, "For me the Ironman is the pinnacle of achievement, it is a far-off goal that takes a lot of work and dedication. It isn't something that you just can do with relative ease, but rather something that requires a total commitment." These triathletes find deep meaning, satisfaction, and joy in setting, working toward, and achieving that goal. Goals inspire, motivate, and fulfill them, not only in triathlon, but in many other parts of their lives.

> *It is blood and guts out there—you are somewhere where you are not in your everyday life. It is a way for us to be tougher, to break the mold, to be whatever you want to be.*
>
> —Nicole DeBoom, pro triathlete

The most common response we received about the benefits of Ironman, which has been echoed numerous times to us by many more triathletes, was the profound love and passion they had for all of its varied and sometimes difficult elements. They also expressed the joy they experienced in so many aspects of their training and race participation. All of the benefits that we described above accumulate to create an experience that, for many people, is deep, enriching, and life altering.

Many Ironman finishers speak of how finishing an Ironman changed their lives. They accomplished something that they never thought was possible. They felt that they were different people who responded to the world in new and better ways. These Ironman triathletes felt inspired, more capable, and ready to tackle life's challenges head-on. Their appreciation of and connection with Ironman was heartfelt and moving.

The Race

The Ironman race itself produces varied emotional reactions from people. Some competitors describe the race as a nonstop joyfest in which they revel in every moment. They love every second from the start of the Ironman training program to the arrival at the race to crossing the finish line. Others describe it as six months and 140.6 miles of hell: the monotony of the training, the fatigue, injuries, and illness, the strained relationships, the apprehension and fear of the swim, the persistent discomfort and boredom of the bike, the painful and seemingly never-ending miles of the marathon.

The roller coaster that is your six months of Ironman training speeds up in the days leading up to your Ironman. All of a sudden, all those hours and miles you've logged are going to be put to the test. You've devoted so much time and energy with no guarantees that your investment will be justified. The dominant emotion felt by many Ironman competitors, including Iron-newbies, seasoned veterans, and pros, is apprehension of the unknown.

Now it's race day and, to paraphrase a famous line, "You ain't felt nothin' yet!" Over the next eight to seventeen hours, you're going to experience the highs and lows of emotion perhaps more frequently and more acutely than ever before in your life. At the swim start, there is a buzz in the air—up to 2,000 Ironman competitors feeling everything from ecstasy to terror. Most likely, you'll feel a mixture of excitement and anticipation at having this moment finally arrive, trepidation at the uncertainty of what lies ahead, and, hopefully, some comfort in knowing that you're prepared to go the distance.

Despite pre-race anxiety, the swim is, in some ways, the easiest because it's the first event, it's short in duration compared to the bike and run, you're well rested, and it's not as physically demanding as the legs to follow. In other ways, the swim is challenging because the open water, mass starts, and the risk of drowning can cause some triathletes to experience apprehension and fear. In either case, the swim, to many, feels long and difficult; you're often faced with physical contact, rough water, and difficulty sighting. Completing the swim is usually a great relief.

When you leave T1, the race really begins. Early in the bike, everyone is settling in; talking and joking with each other, thanking the volunteers and spectators, and feeling good. You may feel mixed emotions at that point: feeling excited to have one event behind you and a sense of wariness knowing that you have a long way to go.

The real challenges of Ironman start to emerge during the last third of the bike. The reality of the race will hit you; you're tired, hungry, thirsty, bored, and hurting—and you still have to run a marathon after the bike. If you go out too fast, you may feel dread knowing the hours of suffering that lie ahead. Many competitors hit the first bottom of the emotional roller coaster between 60 and 90 miles of the bike. Feelings of doubt are common as you begin to tire and more realistically see the task ahead. The emotional roller coaster usually climbs back up during the last 20 miles of the bike. The end of the bike is in sight and, even though a marathon lies ahead, you're just happy to be getting off your bike. You may have a rise in emotions and feel a reinvigoration of energy and renewed confidence, excitement, and motivation.

Watching the run tells you all you need to know about those last hours of an Ironman: most of the field walking, many cramping, some defeated, few happy faces, just a gloomy, yet determined, march to the finish, all in pursuit of completion of a long journey and validation in receiving the Ironman finisher's medal. During the run, the emotional roller coaster dips again. At this point, you'll have been on the course for six to ten hours. You may feel spent and in pain, yet you realize that you still have four to seven more hours on the run. For most, the smiles are long gone and are replaced by a grim look of resolve as competitors plod along, or a desperate look of despair, as some cramp, others hurt, and many question whether they can finish. Many competitors don't feel any particular emotions for most of the run—mainly a numb sense of acceptance that they will be out there for a while and, hopefully, satisfaction that they aren't hurting too much and are still moving along. You also hopefully feel some inspiration because you're seeing your training and race tactics paying off.

The emotional roller coaster changes dramatically as competitors near the athlete village and approach the finish line. The finish is the climactic—and perhaps the most interesting—part of an Ironman. Even after many hours of discomfort and a seemingly empty fuel tank, with the finish within reach, competitors find a store of energy that they may not have known existed. Whether finishing fast in the light of day or walking across in the dark of night, there is an air of unabashed joy and excitement as racers approach the end of their journey. With the finish in sight, most draw on the energy of the roaring crowd, find their legs, and begin to run the last few hundred yards to the finish line. The pain seems to stop briefly and they remember why they chose to do an Ironman. Entering the final stretch, with the crowds cheering, the music blaring, and the announcer screaming, you see finishers jumping with joy, high-fiving spectators, and carrying their children across the finish line. The purity of their elation is inspiring. One first-time Ironman competitor summed it up, "When I heard the announcer say 'Greg B., you are an Ironman,' I realized all the months of effort were so worth being in that moment." For others, the best emotion they can muster is relief that it is finally over. Many Ironman finishers sob uncontrollably, whether for joy, pain, or release we are uncertain.

Ironman racing requires a special mental toughness. Anytime a person is racing for anywhere from eight to seventeen hours, there are going to be a lot of ups and downs mentally. A person needs to be aware of this and know that thinking positively and remembering that things will get better will get you through those low spots.

—Heather Fuhr

But your emotional roller coaster may not stop there. In the weeks of recovery after the race, you will feel a variety of emotions. You hopefully will experience the continued sense of elation and pride in your effort and achievement. If you failed to perform up to your expectations, you may have feelings of frustration and disappointment. You may also experience post-race depression—sadness, listlessness, irritability, and a general malaise—which can come from the physical and psychological letdown that occurs after completion of such a powerful experience (read more on post-race depression in Chapter 7).

With all of the emotions that you experience throughout the Ironman experience, you can be sure that you're not alone in your feelings. Because of the extreme nature of Ironman, intense emotions are the rule rather than the exception and they are part of what make Ironman such an enriching experience. Regardless of what emotions you experience, you can be certain that, in time, they will pass, your life will return to some semblance of normalcy, and now, with experience under your belt, you will have to ask yourself whether it's worth doing another Ironman.

TEN KEYS TO IRONMAN TRAINING

Because training for an Ironman is such a time- and energy-intensive endeavor, the best way to prepare for an Ironman is to know precisely what you will need to do over the next six to nine months and how you will accomplish all of those tasks. The more organized and thorough you are, the more efficient you will be in apportioning out your time and energy, and the more confident you will be that you will have done everything necessary when you arrive at your race.

Have a flexible training plan. When you decide to train for an Ironman, the first thing you should do is make a list of everything you'll need to do to prepare. This list should include a physical training program, equipment, nutrition, mental preparation, lifestyle adjustments, and anything else that you can think of. Because of its complexity, you may not know about or forget an essential piece of the Ironman puzzle. We encourage you to reach out to friends who have done Ironmans, triathlon clubs, coaches, Web sites, books, and magazines to ensure that you have all of your bases covered.

From these diverse resources you can gain a more complete and realistic understanding of what lies ahead in your Ironman efforts. Having gathered this information, you can create a plan that will accommodate everything in the various aspects of your life and allow you to pursue your Ironman goals with full knowledge of what will be required and a plan to do everything that is necessary.

Your Ironman plan must be flexible. As an Iron-newbie, there is no way to predict everything that will happen between the time you sign up for your Ironman and your race. Many aspects of your training and life can change at any point. When changes occur, you should be willing to alter your plan and adapt as needed. By doing so, you'll always be in a position to maximize the time and effort devoted to your Ironman preparations.

Create a quality training program. Having a training program that will enable you to achieve your race goals is the single most important contributor to your Ironman preparations. Your training program should address every area that affects your fitness for the race, including endurance, strength, flexibility, technique, and tactics. The program can include mileage training, interval work, weight training, swim and bike coaching, and nutrition. Of course, it should also address mental areas that will help you through your training and race, such as those discussed in this book.

Because there are so many components to an Ironman training program, we suggest that you seek out a training program from a credible source that you can rely on to get yourself physically ready for the race. In today's triathlon world, you have many available resources to which you can turn to find a quality training program, including local and long-distance one-on-one personal coaching, online coaches, private training teams, local triathlon clubs, books, and charity-based training programs, such as Leukemia and Lymphoma Society Team-in-Training. Having a comprehensive training program will ensure that you arrive at your Ironman safely, well trained, rested, illness- and injury-free, and ready to achieve your goals.

Train smart. As we've mentioned earlier, triathlon training is not about training hard, it's about training smart. Training smart means doing what is necessary to be optimally prepared and striking a healthy balance among frequency, volume, and intensity of training. Most importantly, in the extreme world that is Ironman, training smart means not being seduced by the "more is better" mentality. Being lured into "training stupid" can occur in several ways. You may have training buddies who are training more intensely or who are faster and with whom you want to keep up. Your ego might prevent you from allowing other swimmers, cyclists, or runners to pass you during masters swim sessions, bike hill repeats, or track interval workouts. You may also read, hear about, or see other training programs and think that those programs are better than yours. At the heart of training smart is having confidence that your training program is the best path to your Ironman goals and staying committed to your program in the face of temptations to do more.

Training smart also means training consistently. To gain optimal benefit from your training, you must be consistent in your efforts. This means focus and dedication day after day, week after week, and month after month leading up to your Ironman. A week of high-volume training followed by a few weeks of limited activity, or distance training on the weekends with little to no training during the week, will not allow you to gain the necessary fitness to achieve your Ironman goals and may set you up for injuries. Fitness gains, quality preparation, and Ironman success result from commitment and consistent pursuit of your goals.

Build your confidence progressively. If you commit to doing an Ironman, you may not initially believe you can actually accomplish such an enormous goal. The idea of swimming 2.4 miles, biking 112 miles, and then having to run a marathon may seem simply inconceivable. Well, join the crowd, because most triathletes feel the same way when they decide to train for their first Ironman.

Your lack of confidence is natural given that you don't have experience with that kind of mileage. Your goal, as you prepare for your Ironman, is twofold: to develop the fitness that you need to swim, bike, and run the 140.6 miles and to gain the confidence in your ability to go the distance. Your belief that you can finish is almost as important as having the physical capabilities to do so. Your Ironman training program is about an accumulation of experiences in the pool, on your bike, and in your running shoes, that will incrementally convince you that you can complete an Ironman. With each training milestone—your first 4,000-yard swim, 100-mile bike, and 20-mile run—you gain greater confidence that you can achieve your goal. As we discussed in Chapter 4, your faith in your ability to finish an Ironman will come in small steps from your daily workouts, your ongoing efforts, exposure to adversity, developing essential mental skills, and receiving support and encouragement from others. All of your efforts and preparations will culminate in a level of confidence as you stand at the water's edge before the swim start, and you can say to yourself, "Hey, I can do this!"

Focus on your weaknesses. Contrary to what most people think, you will not achieve your Ironman race goals because of your strengths. Instead, your ability to reach your goals will depend on your weaknesses. The adage, "A chain is only as strong as its weakest link," best describes this relationship. Think of it this way: Even if your strengths begin to break down in the race, they will remain relatively strong, but if your weaknesses break down, they may fail you completely. The more you can develop your weaknesses (and maintain or continue to build your strengths), the more likely you'll cross the finish line.

Particularly early in your training program, direct most of your time and energy to the weakest parts of your Ironman repertoire. If you're a weak swimmer and a strong runner (with cycling somewhere in between), schedule an extra swim workout each week and use that extra time to work on stroke technique and position in the water. Alleviating weaknesses isn't just about more volume. For example, to improve your swimming, you may not only need to get more mileage under your belt, but also gain strength with intervals and weight training, and improve your technique by taking swim lessons.

Keep your training fresh. Beginning an Ironman training program is an exciting and inspiring experience. Early in your Ironman preparations, you'll look forward to your next workout with anticipation. You'll love the newness of your training and enjoy the steady progress you're making. But if you're like many Ironman triathletes, as the weeks and months go by, your initial excitement and enthusiasm may fade as the enormity of the task in front of you becomes more real. At this point, you may be several months into your training program, yet still have months to go. Your mileage is increasing dramatically, and the time and energy you must devote to your training becomes taxing. You may have finally come to see your Ironman in a realistic light, one that is both motivating and stimulating, yet tiring and monotonous as well.

This juncture in your training is crucial because it may determine whether the remaining months leading up to your race are a period of renewed enthusiasm or growing dread for the increasingly arduous challenges awaiting you. You know you've reached this point in your training when you start counting down the weeks before your taper and upcoming workouts cause feelings of trepidation rather than anticipation.

As you cross this line, you may want to step back, perhaps take a few days off, and reconnect with why you chose to pursue an Ironman, the enjoyment you can get out of your training, and the meaning of achieving your goal to finish an Ironman. You may also reevaluate your training, increase your rest days for a few weeks, and look for ways to make your training fresh and interesting. Steps we recommend include training with others rather than alone, reordering your weekly workouts to shake up your routine, changing your training locations, or finding new riding and running routes. You can also learn new ways to accomplish your training goals, such as running on trails rather than roads, doing your running intervals on the road instead of the track, and swimming more often in open water. Modifying your training program in these ways will add novelty and freshness, and will help you stay connected with and continue to enjoy your efforts leading up to your Ironman.

Make recovery a part of your training. Rest and recovery is the most important, yet least emphasized and most often neglected, part of Ironman training. Without proper recovery, your training experience will likely result in overtraining, burnout, illness, or injury. You should incorporate recovery into every level of your training program. On days when you do double workouts, the second should be for recovery. Have a day off structured into your weekly training plan. A recovery week after a two- to three-week high-volume, high-intensity training block is a common part of an Ironman training program. You should include additional, unscheduled recovery days when your body tells you that you need to rest, for example, when you feel unusually tired or ill (for more on recovery, return to Chapter 10).

An essential lesson in Ironman training is to listen to your body. Because you'll be placing incredible demands on your body, you have to respect that it will reach its limits periodically. Your body has a great capacity to communicate with you when it needs a rest (e.g., muscle soreness, fatigue, and illness). It's your responsibility to recognize those signs and respond with adequate recovery time.

Revisit your goals regularly. Just as your Ironman plan is dynamic, your goals should be as well. Work, family commitments, illness, injuries, and unscheduled off days will affect your Ironman preparations. Revisiting and revising your training and race goals each month ensures that you're progressing steadily in your training program. For example, if you miss an important long workout due to a work obligation, shift your training schedule to accommodate the change, or if you're improving faster than anticipated, adjust your training goals to ensure that you continue to be challenged. These revisions to your training program keep your Ironman efforts as focused and effective as possible.

Get a professional bike fit. Perhaps the most arduous part of Ironman training and racing is having to stay in your bike saddle for five to ten hours. As you proceed through the 112-mile ride, your body will become progressively more tired, stiff, and uncomfortable being in the same position for so long. Whether you're able to ride comfortably for hours depends in large part on how well your bike fits your body. A professional bike fitting can ensure that you strike the essential balance between comfort and efficiency.

With miles in the saddle during the months of Ironman training, your body and its fit with the bike will change. As your race approaches, a follow-up fitting can fine-tune your position on the bike and ensure your comfort and efficiency. Though somewhat costly, bike fits are a worthwhile investment for the many hours of training and racing you spend in the saddle.

Make time for the "other" training. Incorporating a mental training program into your Ironman preparations is essential to gaining every advantage as the race approaches. Tracking and adjusting your goals, using positive self-talk and other confidence-building techniques, doing relaxation exercises, developing focus keywords, mastering your emotions, using pain-mastery strategies, and practicing imagery regularly are all vital to your success. Set clear mental training goals each week and incorporate them into your physical training schedule.

TEN KEYS TO IRONMAN SUCCESS

Hopefully, you've arrived at the swim start prepared to finish your Ironman. You put in the training time, and your swim, bike, and run technique is solid. You're mentally prepared to go the distance. But, despite your preparations, there is still no guarantee that you'll be picking up your Ironman finisher's medal later that day. Completing an Ironman is a complex process in which a multitude of things can go wrong. Fortunately, there are a number of steps you can take to minimize the problems that can arise and maximize your chances of having a successful race.

Prepare for the worst. Because of the complexity of an Ironman, competitors rarely have problem-free races. The best way to increase the likelihood that at least most goes well is to prepare for the worst and expect the unexpected. Take preventive measures by figuring out everything that can go wrong and take steps to keep those things from happening. A detailed examination of every aspect of your race can help you identify and respond to potential problem areas. For example, make sure you have your nutritional needs tested in training and dialed in for your race. Inspect all of your equipment—twice. Check the weather and have the proper gear. Have a checklist to ensure that you don't forget anything. And have a plan for each phase of the race including the layout and process of your transitions.

The very nature of Ironman makes the unexpected very likely. Though unforeseen and undesirable occurrences invariably happen during an Ironman, they can just be bumps in the road if you're prepared and you react to them with the right attitude. If you can expect—and plan for—the unexpected, you'll be ready when it occurs, you won't panic, and you'll have a solution for them so you can get back into the race with minimal problems or lost time.

Unexpected events come in all shapes and sizes with varying degrees of irritation and impact on your race. Because Ironman races are so complex and involve so many details, unexpected occurrences often include forgetting essential items (e.g., Greg Bennett, the 2004 ITU world #1, forgot his bike shoes and rode with his running shoes in one Olympic-distance race, and won). Having a list, like the one we provide in

Chapter 11, and double checking it before each phase of your pre-race preparations (e.g., packing for the race, night before, and race morning) will help reduce the likelihood of forgotten gear.

Mechanical failures are frequent in Ironman races; gear problems, loose bolts, and flat tires are the most common. As with most problems, prevention is the best approach. Having your bike tuned before the race and checking beforehand anything that can come loose during a race will minimize their risk of occurrence. You can reduce the chances of a flat by putting on new tires and tubes before your race. But even new tires can get punctures, so carrying several spare tubes and a spare tire, and, most importantly, being skilled at changing tires is essential. A common problem is losing a water bottle from your cage, particularly with seat-post or saddle-mounted cages. We recommend mounting your cages on your frame, as they're easier to reach, and the latest research shows there is no aerodynamic advantage to rear-mounted cages. If you use rear-mounted cages, be sure the cage is high quality and holds the bottles tightly. Jim successfully used a thick rubber band tied to each cage and then wrapped over the nipple of his water bottles at the 2002 Ironman® USA in Lake Placid.

I always thought, what if this happened, how would I deal with it? If I got my goggles knocked off, got kicked in the stomach, if I got a bad time, what would I do? What if I get a flat tire, how do I deal with it? I eliminated all the unknowns by walking through them ahead of time.

—Dave Scott

Changes in weather conditions are typical occurrences in Ironman races, most frequently rain, cold, or heat. Checking the weather report before the race can help you anticipate weather problems. Have the appropriate clothing for weather changes in your transition areas, for example, a rain jacket, long-sleeved jersey, arm warmers for rain and cold, and a cap, sunscreen, and extra liquids for heat and sun. If the changes are particularly serious, carry some of these items on your bike or in a waist pack on the run.

Thorough preparation and planning—paying careful attention to details, identifying things that can go wrong, and taking preventive measures—are the best ways to minimize the chances that something will go wrong during your race. Then, live by the adage, "The best laid plans of mice and men . . ." The reality of Ironman is that no matter what you do to prepare yourself and try to prevent problems from arising, s___ happens.

What will determine whether the bad occurrence ruins your race or is just a bump in the road is your attitude. You can get upset, not solve the problem, and have it end your race. Or you can accept it, find a solution, and get back to the excitement of competing in an Ironman.

Let go of your expectations. The most common question you will be asked before your Ironman is, "What time are you shooting for?" In your naïveté, you may respond, "Well, if all goes well, under X hours." If you answer this question in this way, you're creating two often unrealistic expectations. First is the expectation that all will go well. One of the great lessons we learned about Ironman in particular and triathlon in general is: All rarely goes well. Because of the distance and complexity of an Ironman—equipment, physical demands, logistics, weather—by simple odds, something will go wrong. It's Murphy's Law 140.6-fold for an Ironman. In our discussions with dozens of Ironman finishers, almost none achieved the time goal in their first race and only a few said they have ever had a problem-free race.

Second is the expectation that you can achieve a certain race time that you have set for yourself. Given the vagaries of Ironman, becoming too fixated on a specific finish time can put pressure on you in the days leading up to the race. Time expectations may also cause you to stick to a race plan that isn't working. Our recommendation is to avoid creating expectations over which you have no control.

Expectations can develop in a number of ways. They can arise when you compare yourself to others with whom you train—"If I can keep up with him/her in training, and he/she has done an Ironman in less than thirteen hours, I should be able to do the same." You can also develop unrealistic expectations as you gain fitness and speed in your training. As your confidence in your conditioning builds, so can your expectations. A particularly dangerous way expectations can arise is when you try to extrapolate your training and shorter-race times to your upcoming Ironman—"If I did a 3:00 Olympic distance and a 6:45 half-Ironman, that means I can go under fourteen hours for my Ironman." But speed at shorter distances doesn't necessarily translate into Ironman performance. The mileage that goes into training for an Ironman is more than just multiplying the shorter-distance races by a number until it equals 140.6. The fitness required for an Ironman is more than double that of a half-Ironman.

In our result-driven culture, many triathletes can feel pressure to not only finish—which is a big enough accomplishment—but to finish an Ironman in a certain time. But if you focus too much on the time you want to achieve, it will slowly grow into an "outcome expectation" that you may feel pressure to achieve. This expectation can become a burden and hurt your attitude and effort during the event. Paradoxically, it may also keep you from achieving your time goal. Concentrating on your finish-time expectation will distract you from focusing on executing your race plan and performing your best. Without this focus, the chances of achieving your time expectation are slim.

You may also develop expectations from others. Your family and friends may become invested in your Ironman because they're making sacrifices and want to see their sacrifices justified. They may form an expectation of how you should finish. In a well-meaning, uninformed, and, ultimately, mis-guided attempt at supporting and encouraging you, your supporters may exhort you to achieve a particular time goal without realizing the weight it places on your shoulders.

▼

A lot of it [going fast] has to do with letting go of what you expect and just racing.

—Paula Newby-Fraser

So learn your lesson. When you're asked, "What time are you shooting for?" smile knowingly and say, "I'll give my best effort, I'll execute my race plan, I'll have fun, and I'll finish."

Have a flexible race plan. Competing without a plan is like a warrior going into battle without a strategy to defeat the enemy. Ability and fitness alone aren't enough to go the distance. The best chance you have to achieve your Ironman goals is to have a race plan that guides you from start to finish. This plan involves knowing what you need to do and how and when you need to do it. Your race plan begins the night before the race and concludes when you cross the finish line. It guides you step-by-step through your pre-race activities and leads you through each phase of your race. Before the race, your race plan should include your pre-race fueling, physical warm-up, equipment preparation and inspection, organization of your transition areas, and packing and placement of your special-needs bags.

During the race itself, the important parts of your race plan involve your pacing and fueling. Most competitors use a heart rate monitor and have established heart rate ranges, based on their training efforts, that they want to stay within during the bike and run (it's not possible to monitor your heart rate during the swim). Know precisely the pace and level of exertion you want to maintain during the race. Also, have a well-rehearsed system for your nutrition and hydration needs during each phase of the race.

The single most common cause of Ironman failure is straying from your race plan. You may discard your race plan for a variety of reasons. You may feel so good early in the race that you figure that you can pick up the pace. You may not like to see other competitors passing you and get into a race within the race to keep up. You may stop eating or hydrating according to your plan because your food and drink seem unpalatable. The key is to be disciplined in your approach to the race and not diverge from your plan without a good reason and deliberate consideration.

Though committing to your race plan is important, if it's not working, sticking with it is a recipe for disaster. When your plan isn't working, have a backup plan. There are many variables that can affect your race day, including how you're feeling physically, weather, and course conditions. If any of these factors are influencing you on race day, you may need to alter your race plan. For example, you may need to slow your pace if you're riding into a headwind or drink more if the day is unusually warm. Being able to adjust your race plan when necessary is an essential contributor to a successful Ironman.

> *Always have a Plan B. Plan A is the perfect race, but Plan B is being prepared to be flexible. Keep a calm mind-set and roll with the punches. Be determined to be positive and proactive about what goes on out there.*
>
> —Lance Watson

Having a flexible race plan offers several benefits. Foremost, you have a "method to your madness" during a race. You're not just going out there and hoping to perform well. Rather, you have a plan designed to achieve your goals that will guide you through the race. A race plan also reduces the chances of bad things happening, such as dehydration, cramping, or trying to keep up with other competitors, because your plan tells you precisely what you need to do and what you should avoid. When things do go wrong, you have a backup plan that you count on to keep you moving forward. Having a race plan boosts your confidence, gives you a greater sense of control, and relaxes you because you have a plan that you believe will allow you to have a successful race.

Respect the distance. No matter how much you've trained, if you haven't done an Ironman before, you never quite know what it will be like to swim, bike, and run 140.6 miles. If you've done Ironman races before, you can never anticipate how your next race will go, particularly if you're racing a different course or trying to set a faster time. To achieve your Ironman goals and enjoy the experience, respect the distance. This appreciation for the challenges that the distance presents will ensure that you stay within yourself during the race and don't think you have it made until you see the finish chute in sight.

Anyone who has raced in the paralyzing heat and energy-sapping wind of the Ironman® World Championships in Hawaii quickly learns the futility of trying to beat the course. One experience on any Ironman course is a powerful reality check on the absurdity of trying to defeat the terrain or the elements. Ironman competitors quickly learn that the best they can hope to do is accept and adapt to the course, for example, easing their cycling effort into a headwind or slowing their run pace in 95-degree weather. Successful Ironman triathletes understand that every competitor faces the same course on race day, so it isn't the course that matters, but whether they respect the course and how they react to what lies ahead.

I wanted to finish because I wanted to be embarrassed. It's a very embarrassing thing when you're walking and people are tapping you on the bum, saying, "Come on Macca." I wanted to go through it all; I wanted to suffer and take that with me into my training for next year.

—Chris McCormack

No better example of the need to respect the distance can be found than in Australian Chris McCormack, widely viewed as the top short-course triathlete in recent years. After dominating Olympic-distance and half-Ironman races, he moved up to Ironman-distance races in 2002 and won his first, Ironman® Australia. Entering the 2002 World Championships in Hawaii, Macca, as he is known, was considered a favorite for the title and spoke with what some characterized as bravado and arrogance about his chances of victory. Macca came off the bike near the lead, but bonked a few miles into the run and didn't finish. In 2003, with similar expressions of confidence and expectations of victory, he was once again among the leaders entering T2, but he bonked early in the run and only finished by walking much of the run course. When the 2004 World Championships were approaching, Macca expressed a newfound humility for Kona and a healthy respect for the distance (and yet he didn't finish).

Fuel consistently. A common cause of Ironman failure is poor nutrition. Because your body needs fuel regularly throughout your Ironman, you must be diligent and disciplined in eating and drinking at regular intervals. You will have two primary obstacles to staying well nourished. First, you may simply forget. You can get so wrapped up in the race that fueling slips your mind. This forgetfulness is exacerbated by the fact that you need to eat and drink before you're hungry or thirsty, so you don't always receive cues from your body that remind you to eat or drink until it's too late. Many Ironman competitors arrange for reminders during the race, for example, placing a piece of tape that reads "EAT" on their handlebars or setting their watch timer to ring at set intervals.

Second, late in an Ironman, food and drink can become entirely unpalatable. Taking another bite of an energy bar, squeezing another bit of gel into your mouth, or taking another sip of your energy drink can be a truly aversive experience. If you can't put it in your mouth, any nutritional value your fuel has becomes moot. We suggest that palatability, assuming reasonable nutritional value, should be a dominant factor in choosing your Ironman race food and drink. Ironman veterans we know swear by peanut butter and jelly sandwiches, Fig Newtons, and Pop-Tarts as race-food choices. Having a variety of foods and a combination of sweet and salty tastes also helps with both nutritional needs and palatability. Drinks are more difficult to choose because they provide Ironman triathletes with most of their calories, and many of the well-known energy drinks are dense and not particularly flavorful. Just like your food, the energy drink you choose should be tested during long training rides and runs. Be sure that you like how it tastes after hours of exertion and, importantly, when it's warm. During the run, aid stations offer more varieties of fuel, mostly "normal" food, such as bananas, candy bars, and chicken broth, so you have the opportunity to offer your rebellious taste buds something new and better tasting. Whatever keeps you from eating and drinking sufficiently, remain alert to the need to fuel regularly and commit to eating and drinking whether you want to or not.

Keep your self-talk positive. In Chapter 4, we discussed the value of positive self-talk for triathlon success. It plays an even more dramatic role in an Ironman. At about 80 miles of the bike, the point at which most Ironman veterans will tell you the race really begins, your body will start to break down. The farther you get in the race, the more your energy will wane, even though your training has given you the fitness to make it to the finish. What you say to yourself during the remaining 60.6 miles will be the key to achieving your Ironman goals.

Staying positive during the later stages of an Ironman is critical. Keeping your self-talk positive starts by consistently practicing this skill in training when your body is hurting and your attitude is being challenged. The more you can train yourself to stay positive in training, the more likely you will keep positive in your race. During the race, regularly monitor your attitude, and if it starts to deteriorate, recognize the need for an attitude adjustment or an infusion of calories. The need for positive self-talk is most important late in the race when your body is breaking down and you're in considerable pain. An ongoing internal monologue of positive statements that reminds you of your goal and how good it will feel to realize your dream of being an Ironman can make the difference in the race. Positive self-talk reminds you why you're tolerating the discomfort, distracts you from the pain, and generates positive emotions that help ease your pain and motivate you to overcome it.

Have a focus. One of your biggest challenges during your Ironman is maintaining your focus throughout the race. Because the race is so long, you may have difficulty paying attention to everything that's important. Additionally, you'll be faced with many distractions that pull your focus away from the race, for example, other competitors, scenery, volunteers and spectators, physical discomfort, and your time goal. The most important focus to have during the race is on the process and what you can control in the present. If you focus on the here and now (e.g., swim stroke, breathing, fueling, pace, etc.), you'll perform your best and you'll be less stressed about the fact that you may be out there for a long time.

> *To be mentally focused you need to talk to yourself a lot! Of course, you can't be focused 100 percent of the time, but when you start to find yourself daydreaming or dwelling on the pain, you have to make a good effort to think positive thoughts and concentrate on other things.*
>
> —Lori Bowden

Before the race you can help your focus by identifying everything you need to concentrate on at different points in the race. Though an Ironman is a complicated endeavor, you want to focus on the essentials and reduce your focus on nonessentials. As we discussed above, pace and fueling may be your two most important concerns during the race. Focusing on your heart rate, form, and nutrition as priorities sets you up well for a successful day.

You can also identify specific cues on which you want to focus at different stages of the race. For example, during the swim, your focus might include not going out too fast at the start, settling into a good rhythm early, and steering clear of other swimmers. On the bike, your focus could consist of fueling regularly, changing your body position periodically, and monitoring the lactic acid buildup in your legs. For the run, your focus might include staying relaxed, continuing to eat and drink at aid stations, and listening to your body to make adjustments in your pace, stride, and posture.

Developing keywords or phrases is a useful tool to help you remember your focus for different parts of the race. For the swim, "keep it cool," "smooth stroke," and "free water" would be effective reminders. During the bike, "fuel up," "stretch out," and "spin" would be helpful. On the run, "swing the arms," "drink and eat up," and "talk to the body" would be useful reminders.

Finally, it's both impossible and unnecessary for you to be continually focused on your race from start to finish. As we mentioned in Chapter 6, taking your mind off the race can be a useful and liberating strategy. During the bike and run, thank the volunteers and spectators, talk to other riders, and look at the scenery. But don't drift off too often or for too long. You might miss some valuable information. Always keep monitoring yourself and refocus on the race when necessary.

> *The race is about dealing with everything, from traveling to setting up your bike to preparing yourself mentally. And that mental preparation involves keeping focused. If something goes wrong, don't blow up; put your energy into fixing it. You have to deal with it and move on, because something else will happen—it always does.*
>
> —Peter Reid

Use your mental toolbox. Your training program gave you the physical capabilities to go the distance in your Ironman, but it will be how well trained your mind is that determines whether you cross the finish line. Hopefully, you put in time on your mental training and put a variety of mental tools in your toolbox during your Ironman preparations that you can use in the race. As any Ironman will tell you, as the race progresses, it becomes less physical and more mental. At this point, you want to be able to reach into your mental toolbox and access specific mental tools when necessary.

Mental tools that you'll need include motivational cues to keep you going when you're hurting, self-talk to help you stay positive, relaxation exercises to keep loose, keywords to remain focused, emotional mastery strategies to help maintain control, and pain-management techniques to keep you going when your body is telling you to stop. Being aware of the mental tools you bring to the race and having the wherewithal to open your toolbox during the race will enable your mind to keep your body moving toward the finish line late in the race when it starts to fall apart.

Recover from down periods. An inevitable part of doing an Ironman is that you will experience down periods during your race. These bad spells may be caused by a nutritional crisis, pain, fatigue, or the emotional challenges of covering 140.6 miles. They usually occur at between 60 and 90 miles of the bike and near the midpoint of the run. An essential lesson to learn is that these down periods are not bottomless pits without hope of recovery and they do not have to end your race.

A down period is a warning signal that your body or mind is becoming distressed. These declines are experienced as a decrease in energy, loss of motivation, a growing negative attitude, and an increase in negative emotions, such as frustration or despair. You want to recognize them as early as possible, before you descend too far into the abyss. Once you see you're heading down a bad road, you can do something about it. When you start to feel yourself slipping downward, check your heart rate (if you're wearing a monitor). You may be outside your aerobic zone and need to adjust your pace. Inadequate nutrition is the most common cause of these bad spells. At the earliest signs of a down period, take in extra fuel. The bad spell may be from the emotional toll that you incur during an Ironman. When your emotions begin to turn negative, deliberately focusing on positive and motivating self-talk, staying relaxed, and generating positive emotions can turn the tide on the bad spell. More than anything, believing that you can recover from down periods will help you not become overwhelmed by the bad feelings, maintain perspective on the bad spells—"I can get over this"—and give you the fortitude to actively reverse the downward path you are on.

Revel in the experience. The ultimate reason you should do an Ironman is because you enjoy the Ironman experience. During your training,

> *Know that a race like an Ironman is a long day and that you will have ups and downs throughout the day. Get through the tough parts and really enjoy the good parts.*
>
> —Pete Kain

celebrate your increasing fitness, being outdoors, the people you swim, ride, and run with, and the physical and mental challenges you surmount. At the race, enjoy the athlete village, meeting and swapping stories with new and veteran Ironman competitors, exploring the course, and making your final preparations. During the race, reveling in the jump-with-joy sense of the word may not be possible given the physical demands you'll be placing on yourself and the ongoing discomfort you will feel. Nonetheless, take the time to appreciate the opportunity you've given yourself, the volunteers and spectators, and the shared challenges. After you've crossed the finish line, revel completely in your successful journey, the excitement of achieving a monumental goal, and sharing your joy with family, friends, and other Ironman finishers.

> *I was ecstatic coming across the finish line. It was almost like I'd won the race.*
>
> —Peter Reid

A HUMOROUS (THOUGH REALISTIC) VIEW OF A FIRST-TIME IRONMAN

An Ironman will be, for the six months that you train for it, the sole focus and guiding force in your life. You will spend many hours each week training for Ironman. You will spend even more hours each week thinking, dreaming, talking, and reading about Ironman. Ironman will consume you.

Your life will revolve around training (up to twenty hours a week), sleeping (going to bed by 9:00 P.M. and getting up before dairy farmers and West Coast stockbrokers), food (you can and want to eat everything in sight), and drink (you will have seven or more forms of liquid in your fridge). Your social life will involve 5:00 A.M. masters swims, Saturday rides, and Sunday runs. If you're married, have children, or have friends who are not triathletes, heaven help them! You will be thankful that you're single or have a forgiving partner. Or you'll become a skilled negotiator, willing to concede anything and everything (e.g., "I'll take out the garbage for the next year") for that extra hour of riding on Saturday.

Your conversations will revolve around your past triathlon experiences, your training program, and your race goals. You will ask everyone who has ever done an Ironman for training and race tips, and then you will obsess over which of the always-conflicting tips you should accept. You will ask essential life questions, such as "Is an online coach worth it?" "Will an aero seat post make me faster?" and "Is the swim that important?" You will be faced with major life decisions: goggles or mask; carbon, aluminum, or steel; 73° or 78°; 700s or 650s?

You will become a voracious and insatiable consumer of all things Ironman: training, equipment, technique, nutrition, fashion. You will subscribe to and read cover-to-cover all of the tri-mags. You will buy videos on swim technique. You will attend lectures given by the world's best triathletes and coaches and grill them with questions after. You will surf the Internet finding the most obscure Web sites devoted to Ironman and savor every new morsel of information you consume. You will look forward to going to your local tri-store hoping there is something you forgot to buy that you absolutely must have. You will make lists of what you will need in your Ironman, what you will put in each transition and special-needs bag, and what you will have to do the day before and the day of the race. You will call the top pros by their nicknames—"Hey, Macca, Walto!"

You will live for your daily workouts. You will have trouble falling asleep because you can't wait to get up the next day and train. You will compulsively record every detail of your training program in your computer: distance, time, heart rate, splits, strokes per length, miles per hour, minutes per mile. You will track your progress. You will wonder how a person can enjoy swimming 100 laps in a 21.88-yard pool and riding a bike for seven hours, and then you will understand how. You will revel in completing your first 2-mile swim, 100-mile ride, and 20-mile run. You will add "brick" to your vocabulary and use it proudly. You will add up your weekly volume every Sunday and gush with pride as you approach twenty hours.

You will develop a deep and abiding hatred of water bottles. You will have at least ten water bottles at some point in a never-ending cycle of Ironman life: on your bike, in the sink soaking with soapy water, in the dish rack drying, or taking up an entire counter in your kitchen, poised, seemingly eager, to return to your bike.

You will arrive late to work, take long lunch breaks, and leave early. You will fall asleep at your desk. You will fantasize about being able to train full-time. You will pray that you have a forgiving boss or be thankful you are your own boss. You will not get fired. Your body will look different—leaner, more muscular, harder. You will walk differently: a new spring in your step, a bit of swagger in your gait. You will feel differently—tired, yet energized, relaxed, yet jazzed. You will think differently: more confident, determined, and focused. After never having experienced the runner's high, you will get the "tri-high" regularly. You will begin to think training is better than sex.

You will experience more emotional highs and lows in one day than you usually feel in a week. You will feel excitement, frustration, hope, despair, doubt, awe, sadness, and inspiration, and that's before you've even left for your 100-mile ride. You will constantly question why you are doing an Ironman—and you will come up with different answers every time. You will dream of qualifying for Kona, even if the only chance you have is to win the lottery. You will smile with joy at the thought of being an Ironman and cringe in fear at the thought of not finishing.

At the start of the race, you'll pray you don't get trampled in the swim mass start. You'll run through the transitions hoping to save an extra thirty seconds. From miles 60–90, you will swear to give your bike away as soon as you get home, yet feel like you're on a pleasure ride the last 20 miles. Your energy drink and solid food you brought on the bike will become absolutely unpalatable. You will never know such joy as riding into T2, until you realize that you still have to run 26.2 miles. For the first 20 miles, you will finally understand the adage, "Misery loves misery's company." You will never want to see another energy bar or gel again. You'll realize that chicken soup really is food for the soul. You will feel muted satisfaction at the people you pass and great trepidation at those who pass you. From miles 20 to 24, you will wonder what you were thinking when you decided to do an Ironman. With 2 miles to go, whether running or walking, you will find a reservoir of energy that you never knew was there. Catching sight of the finish will be like approaching the Pearly Gates of heaven. And, after 140.6 miles, for just a few moments, you will feel light as a feather as you cross the finish line.

After the race, you will feel like you are about to explode with pride and you will sob uncontrollably. You'll swear never to do another Ironman, then sign up for one two weeks later. You won't want to take off your finisher's medal. You will look forward to wearing all of that overpriced, yet oh-so-worth-it, Ironman clothing that you bought at the expo. You will revel in taking a few weeks off after the race and being a total slug. Then the itch to return to training will slowly creep up on you. Your first workout back you will feel different: stronger, tougher, the real deal. You will savor wearing the hat or shirt that announces to the world that you are an Ironman. You will feel special, like you've joined an exclusive club. You can now say, "I am an Ironman."

TRIATHLETE SPOTLIGHT: JENNY

Jenny, a 33-year-old, learned the lesson of expectations at the 2002 Ironman® USA in Lake Placid. Having been a runner, she never felt the slightest bit of anxiety before her eight previous marathons. But in the days leading up to Lake Placid, she was very nervous. She felt awful physically, was not enjoying her Ironman experience, and was not looking forward to the race. She was looking for some excuse to not have to race.

At the heart of her angst was the pressure she felt to achieve her time expectation and a persistent fear that she would go out too hard, bonk early, and have many hours of self-inflicted suffering. Two days before the race, she called her coach and told him how she felt. He said that her feelings were natural because she had chosen to undertake an enormous challenge and that the best way to let go of the anxiety was to let go of her time expectations. He told Jenny to set three goals: enjoy herself, maintain a comfortable pace, and finish strong.

As soon as he suggested this, Jenny felt like a huge weight had been lifted from her shoulders. In the final forty-eight hours, she had fun and felt excited about the race. Before the race, she decided to take her coach's advice to the extreme. The night before the race, she taped over her bike computer so she wouldn't see her bike time, miles per hour, or the miles she was covering. She also didn't start her stopwatch at the beginning of the race. During almost the entire race, she had no idea how fast she was going or how long she was on the course. In fact, she didn't think about her race time until well into the marathon.

By freeing herself of her time expectation, Jenny relieved herself of the pressure to achieve it when just finishing an Ironman was sufficiently daunting and accomplishment enough. Instead, she focused on her race plan. In the swim, she concentrated on not getting pummeled in the mass start, staying relaxed, maintaining good form, and conserving her energy. On the bike, she paid attention to her pace, riding conservatively and making sure she stayed in her aerobic zone. Heading out on the run, she felt so good she actually had to hold herself back. At mile 19, she was feeling so strong that she decided to let herself go. She attacked the last 7 miles and finished in a rush and on a high. And, guess what? She achieved her time goal—less than thirteen hours—to boot!

15 Tips from the Top

Through our triathlon and sport psychology experiences, and interviews with some of the finest triathletes in the world, we've compiled a series of "tips from the top" (thanks to Dave Scott, Mike Pigg, Heather Fuhr, Paul Huddle, Pete Kain, and Victor Plata). These valuable lessons can help you raise your performances and achieve your triathlon goals regardless of your age, ability, or aspirations.

Trust your preparation. Learning to trust your preparation is one of the biggest challenges you face. You never know with 100-percent certainty whether your preparation is adequate until you've tested your fitness in a race, but you can develop trust in your preparation as the race approaches. This faith in your readiness comes from seeing progress in different aspects of your conditioning. Trust also builds from workouts that test your fitness and simulate race distance and intensity, for example, a 30-mile bike and 5-mile run brick for an Olympic-dis-

> *I remember how bad my legs felt. I couldn't think of racing for a while; my legs felt dreadful. I had to remind myself that I've had lots of runs like this, lots of training like this. . . . I had to shift to remembering and confidence.*
>
> —Dave Scott

tance race. You can also gain trust in your preparation for a big race by racing in other events and seeing your fitness pay off.

Trust in your preparation acts as the foundation for achieving your race goals. It enables you to execute a realistic race plan. Trust allows you to push your limits because you know where your limits are. It gives you the confidence and motivation to keep going when you go through a rough patch during a race, knowing that you have the fitness to recover. You're able to recall the time and energy you devoted to your preparations and know that it can carry you through the difficult parts of the race.

It is important to figure out a mental approach that suits your personality. While it may be fine for someone to do mental imagery, others may need to take an approach that is more "go with the flow" or in the now.

—Heather Fuhr

Personalize your mental approach to racing. Just as you customize your physical training program to fit your personality—for example, you can train alone or with a group, or you may prefer working out in the mornings or evenings—you should also develop a mental approach that suits your personality. If you are highly organized in all things triathlon, a similar structure to your mental preparation may be appropriate. This methodical approach, not unlike your conditioning program, might include developing and implementing the goal-setting and mental training program we describe in Chapter 9 with a well-thought-out calendar of mental training techniques and strict adherence to the schedule.

If, however, you tend toward a "do it as I feel it" attitude to the sport, a more spontaneous approach to your mental training may be best. This lack of structure might involve using various mental training strategies as the need arises naturally. For example, you might use relaxation exercises on your shoulders when you feel them tense during a run or positive self-talk during a ride when you notice yourself being negative. Regardless of the approach you take, mental training will only have value if you do it consistently. Taking a consistent mental approach that fits with your personality will likely result in greater enjoyment in mental training, continued use, and optimal benefit.

Expect to feel nervous. Prime Triathlon is about performing your best in the most important races of your life. It may be your first triathlon, your first half-Ironman, or your first chance at a Kona slot. You may start to feel nervous as the race approaches. This reaction is common among triathletes at all levels of ability; it happens to age groupers, and it happens to the best triathletes in the world. Much of this book is directed toward helping you achieve prime intensity and avoid pre-race anxiety. The reality is, though, that getting nervous before important races is normal and natural. One way to partially alleviate the negative effects of too much intensity is to expect to be nervous. Anticipate experiencing some anxiety before the race, so when it arises your reaction will be, "This is normal. I knew I would get a little nervous. No big deal."

Anxiety can also be interpreted in different ways producing very different reactions. If you view anxiety as negative and threatening, it can hurt your performance. If you see it, instead, as an indication that you're getting yourself psyched up for a big race, then you'll interpret the feeling positively. With a more positive perspective on the added intensity, you can then use the psych-down techniques we discussed in Chapter 5 to take the edge off your nervousness and allow you to feel more comfortable. Another important realization is that whatever you're feeling, many others around you are likely feeling the same way. Even if they look cool, calm, and collected on the outside, chances are they're equally as nervous on the inside, further affirming that some anxiety is to be expected.

Expect it to be difficult. Triathlons are difficult. You do triathlons because they're physically demanding and because they stretch you mentally. Races test your physical, technical, tactical, and mental capabilities. They show you what you're made of mentally and emotionally, requiring you to muster motivation, confidence, intensity, focus, and emotions in pursuit of your goals. They place your body under extreme stress, which affirms your fitness. The greater the challenges during the race, the more fulfillment, excitement, and elation you'll feel after the race.

If you expect it to be difficult, you'll prepare yourself physically and mentally for the demands of the race. You'll put in the time swimming, biking, and running so that when it gets tough, your body and mind will respond positively. If you expect it to be grueling, then there won't be any surprises, just acceptance and a positive reaction. If you're really hurting, that's part of the experience. If you're having a bad day, that

Some days you have to fight and fight and fight for every meter. And today was like that.

—Nicole Leder,
2002 Ironman® Brazil champion

happens. If you give your best effort and you still don't achieve your goals, you can still take pride in having given it your all.

Be patient. Patience is an essential quality for achieving your triathlon goals. It plays an important role in your training and race efforts. Your ability to control your urges to push ahead in training and races can determine the progress of your fitness, your race readiness, and your race-day performance.

Patience must begin in training. Strength, stamina, and flexibility can't be rushed. You must allow these components of your fitness to develop through your ongoing and progressive training efforts. As we've discussed earlier, patience is expressed by a balance of training frequency, volume, intensity, and recovery. Patience can prevent training setbacks, such as overtraining, illness, and injury, all of which will slow your progress. Asserting patience in your training involves sticking to your program, maintaining a long-term perspective on your progress, training at your own predetermined pace, keeping your ego in check during workouts, and actively controlling your impatient impulses. Patience is a skill that develops with practice. You can work on your patience during masters swim workouts, on group rides, and in track workouts.

Staying patient in your training will prepare you to be patient in races. Patience in races acts as a governor when you're feeling unusually good, getting overeager, not wanting others to pass you, or not appreciating the distance. It can prevent you from going at an unrealistic pace, maintaining an effort above your anaerobic threshold, and bonking later in the race. Staying patient in your races means having and adhering to a clear race plan, respecting the distance, keeping the late stages of the race in mind, and recognizing that all of your early efforts are aimed at conserving energy for late in the race and a strong finish.

> *Yesterday was definitely a mental day because of the winds. That's when all the training in the world doesn't matter. You have to tell yourself to keep going, be patient, and never give up.*
>
> —Natasha Badmann,
> four-time Ironman world champion

You can't always be "on." The odds are that you'll have one or more races during triathlon season in which you're not "on." You may not be on top of your game due to fatigue, illness, injury, life stress, or any number of reasons. You may begin a race and just not feel good, and know you're not going to achieve your race goals.

You can't always perform at 100 percent, but even with an off day, if you adjust your goals, you can still have a valuable and enjoyable experience. Your overall goal should be to continue to give your best effort and perform as well as you can on that day. More specifically, when you realize that you're not going to have a good race, step back from your initial disappointment and ask yourself what good can come of it. When you find something positive that you can get out of your race—and something good can come from the worst race experiences—focus on that benefit and direct your energy toward achieving that goal. After the race, ask yourself what you learned, how you could have prepared better, and what you can do differently at your next race.

Having an off day is an opportunity to overcome internal adversity. Prevailing over weather and course conditions is difficult and satisfying, but overcoming yourself is even more challenging and rewarding. Races where you're not on form are great occasions to simply enjoy your race experience, for example, the scenery, the people, and the chance to be outdoors. This means giving up any performance expectations you have. Off days also allow you to work on some part of your race that you wouldn't ordinarily focus on, such as your body position on the bike or your posture on the run.

Respond quickly to challenges. Prime Triathlon is based on the notion of performing at a consistently high level under the most challenging conditions. However, performing consistently does not mean that you will not have problems or experience declines in races. One thing that makes the world's best triathletes so good is not that they don't struggle during races, but rather how they respond to the challenges they do face and how quickly they recover. Races are often made or lost on who can recover from their difficulties most quickly.

Recovering from challenges quickly begins with an accepting attitude in which you allow that you will have difficulties and understand that negative reactions will only hurt the situation. Accepting problems as part of triathlon makes it easier for you to let go of them. With the negative impact of difficulties reduced, direct your attention to getting yourself back physically and mentally. Maintain your confidence and keep your self-talk positive. Redirect your focus onto the process and the present, in other words, what you need to do to resolve the problem and regain your form. Check and adjust your intensity to ensure your body is relaxed and ready to perform well again.

Having dealt with the mental and emotional aspects of the difficulty, directly address the problem at hand. Recognize and identify the problem, whether physical, technical, tactical, or related to the conditions, as soon as possible. Then solve the problem by making an adjustment, and focus on the solution in the immediate future.

Keep it simple. Triathlon is, in some ways, a complex sport. There is an overwhelming amount of information about triathlon in magazines, books, and online. You have to train for three different disciplines. You must buy and maintain all sorts of equipment and gear. You have to learn about and use many types of nutritional products. You need to coordinate the complicated logistics that exist in every triathlon. There are expectations from friends and family, and, for the pros, sponsors and the media. And you must adhere to a multifaceted race plan and respond to the many unexpected events that arise during a triathlon. It's easy to get caught up in all this minutiae and lose sight of the heart of triathlon.

Triathlon is, at its core, a simple sport. You devote the time and energy to prepare yourself completely. You give your best effort. You dig deep when things get tough. And you hang in there until you cross the finish line. You may think that the pros are successful because they've mastered the complexities of triathlon, but we've learned that they're so accomplished because of their emphasis on the sport's most basic elements.

When you begin to feel overwhelmed by triathlon life, remind yourself of the basics of the sport. Training should be challenging and enjoyable. The people should be interesting and fun. Races should be difficult and rewarding. Jettison the excess baggage of triathlon and remember that triathlon is made up of three events that you loved to do as a child, and

> *It's really a simple thing. It's your outlet in life. You train, rest, and race. That's what it amounts to. We can start to complicate things more than is needed. Try and let go of some of the minutiae and big issues and just focus on the simple things. Control what you can and let go of what you can't. It's really not much more complicated than that.*
> —Paul Huddle

you are now fortunate enough to "play" again. Focusing on the simplicity of the sport enables you to regain your motivation and confidence, relax, and reconnect with what attracted you to triathlon in the first place.

Learn from your setbacks. Whether you're a tri-newbie, an age grouper, or a pro, you will experience fatigue, pain, boredom, overtraining, illness, injury, equipment failure, poor race conditions, bad tactics, unrealized expectations, and many other setbacks in your training and racing. How you react to the setbacks will determine how they affect your future training efforts, race performances, and enjoyment of the sport. For setbacks to be beneficial, you should view them as opportunities to learn lessons that will foster your development as a triathlete and growth as a person.

Learning from your setbacks begins with accepting them as normal parts of life. This acknowledgment lessens their shock value and reduces your emotional reaction to them. Have a positive attitude toward the setback, maintaining your confidence and motivation to continue to move forward. Find a solution to the setback that resolves it in the present and also teaches you a lesson about how to prevent and respond to it in the future. Finally, put the setback behind you and focus on what you need to do to continue the pursuit of your goals.

> *You learn the most from your setbacks. They test your character, and when you get through them, you come back stronger than before.*
> —Siri Lindley

Race experience is invaluable. There is simply no substitute for race experience in becoming a consistently successful triathlete. You can put in yards in the pool, miles on the bike, and laps on the track, attend lectures, read magazines, and watch videos, but none of these experiences can duplicate the logistical, physical, tactical, mental, and emotional demands of a race. The race is the ultimate classroom to learn about triathlon.

Training allows you to build a foundation for achieving your race goals. It provides you with the opportunity to gain general knowledge about the volume, intensity, and frequency you need to achieve your race goals. You can test your hydration and fueling. You're able to experiment with technique, body position, and pace. And you can fine-tune these areas as the race approaches. But what works in training doesn't always work in races. You'll never know if various aspects of your preparations are effective until you put them to the test in a race.

The reality is that no matter how great your effort is in training, it cannot approach the physical and mental challenges of a race. Race experience offers you a unique setting in which to learn about what you need to do to achieve your goals. It differs from training because it matters, it counts, there will be a public record of your performance. In most cases, a race will be the first time that you put all three disciplines together. It will also be the first time that your body is faced with the pace, intensity, and discomfort of competition. Race experience allows your body to become accustomed and adapt to those physical demands. It allows your mind to become familiar with the challenges to motivation, confidence, intensity, focus, emotions, and pain that you will face. It provides you with a real-world "laboratory" in which to test your equipment and nutritional strategies under race conditions. Most powerfully, race experience exposes your weaknesses in ways that can't be ignored. Repeated exposure to these race experiences enables you to become familiar and comfortable with these demands, learn what you're capable of and what you need to work on, and to develop strategies to cope with the challenges.

> *The thing that made me mentally tough was experience and putting myself in race situations. It takes a bunch of times getting beat to become a champion. You have to go out there and get the experience. Don't worry about winning or losing; you're not going to learn how to win until you race. You have to toe up if you really want to learn.*
>
> —Mike Pigg

We recommend that you gain experience in all types of races: short and long, hot and cold, flat and hilly, small and big. Having diverse race experiences will expose you to a wider range of conditions, obstacles, and challenges. From these experiences, you'll gain more knowledge and skills that you can apply to your training and future race challenges. You'll also have more tools in your toolbox and be able to adapt to more diverse race situations.

Take time to rest your mind. The life of a triathlete can be busy and stressful. You have work, time with family and friends, and other personal interests, in addition to the time and energy you devote to your triathlon training and racing. A structured part of most training programs is physical rest following an intense training period and a taper before a race. The purpose of both is to give your body the time to recover and recharge. But little thought is given to resting the mind and giving it the opportunity to recover from training and prepare for a race. Yet a tired mind can be as harmful to race success as a tired body.

Resting your mind allows you to put the intensity of training behind you and gain a fresh and excited perspective about the race. A rested mind will be more confident and positive, particularly in the challenges you'll face during the race, and it will be better able to stay focused on the race and avoid distractions. A rested mind will be more resilient to race stress and less likely to respond with frustration and despair.

How you rest your mind is up to you. If you have the luxury of taking a few days off from work or school before your race, that is very restful. In the absence of that kind of flexibility, you can read a book, listen to music, watch a movie, go for a walk, or spend time with family or friends—anything that is relaxing and takes your mind off stressors related to life or your race.

> *We need to rest our minds to get the fire going for the race. Part of my success was that I was good at resting my mind. A lot of good athletes out there should have beaten me in races, and they either didn't rest their bodies or they didn't rest their minds. That clean, rested mind, as a muscle, will be ready to give 100 percent on race day.*
>
> —Mike Pigg

Accept the challenge. As we discussed in Chapter 7, a significant obstacle to performing your best and realizing your triathlon goals is fear. Fear produces a cautious attitude and a tentative effort. When fear controls you, your primary goal is to play it safe and hope to not fail rather than expect to succeed. You don't perform aggressively, take risks, or push your limits. There are few things more unsatisfying than going down with a whimper, rather than a bang.

Before a race, accept the challenge to perform with courage and the willingness to risk in order to achieve your goals. Resolve to compete to your fullest ability. Commit to doing everything you can to perform your best. Accept that when you have this attitude, you still may not reach your goals. Understand that you can't control the course, weather, or your

When you are out there racing in the heat, a lot of doubts come into your head. The kahunas were telling me I had to have the courage to go through the race and win. But first I must be brave.

—Mark Allen

result, but you can control the effort you put in and how you respond to challenges you will face. If you accept the challenge and compete with commitment and resolve, then you're much more likely to perform your best and feel good about your race.

TRIATHLETE SPOTLIGHT: JAKE

Jake, a 26-year-old who was in his first year of doing triathlons, seemed to make things difficult for himself. His first three races of the season were a jumble of nerves, naïveté, and race problems. Having been a high school star in several team sports, Jake expected the transition to triathlon to be easy. He was frustrated because he figured he'd be beating most of the other guys in his tri-club and challenging for the podium immediately. But at each race, there were other competitors who weren't nearly as good of athletes as he was, but who were passing him left and right.

Being an excitable guy, Jake would become so absorbed with the race in the week leading up to it that he could think about little else. He would get himself so amped that he would sleep poorly leading up to the race and would be exhausted on race morning.

He also couldn't believe that so many things could go wrong in a race. He would get upset when a problem arose; for example, in two of his races, he had a flat (which took him forever to fix) and lost two water bottles, respectively. After each incidence of bad luck, it took him awhile to clear his head and get back into the race.

Jake attended a talk given by a sport psychologist at a local sports store and saw that he was really shooting himself in the foot in his triathlon efforts. He first admitted that triathlon was actually different from the team sports he played in high school and that his natural ability wasn't enough to be successful. Though he trained pretty hard, he hadn't been swimming or biking for very long, and he realized that he needed to be patient and allow his fitness to develop.

Jake learned that his excitement before races, unlike for football and basketball games, hurt his performance. He needed to relax and conserve energy heading toward race day. If he wanted to arrive at the race rested and with a good mind-set, he needed to "chill out." In the days before the race, he kept himself busy and kept his mind off of the race. He listened to relaxing music and took a hot bath on the two nights before his race. He slept much better leading up to the race.

At one of his tri-club's meetings, Jake asked one of its veteran members about his problems on race day. He laughed and said, "Welcome to triathlon." Jake learned that races are rarely problem free, and he should expect at least one thing to go wrong and to not sweat it; just deal with it and move on. He should figure out everything that can go wrong and make a plan for handling it. In the weeks before the race, he practiced changing his tires several times until he could do it with minimal trouble. He also bought new cages that held his water bottles better.

Jake woke up on race morning feeling rested and ready to go. He got himself organized and reminded himself that his goal was to have a good, consistent race and not worry about his time or who he might beat. He continued to focus on staying relaxed in the time leading up to the start. Late in the bike, he got a flat (he was almost hoping to get one), but he didn't get upset about it. Patting himself on the back for having practiced tire changes, he quickly replaced the flat and was on his way again before he knew it. He told himself that he couldn't change the past, so he immediately refocused on finishing the bike strong and having a good run.

Jake finished on a high, pleased with his performance. He was amazed at how a few changes in his mind-set and approach to triathlon had made a big difference in his attitude toward the race and how well he did. He was now ready to really commit himself to triathlon and to see how fast he could go.

CHAPTER

16 Embracing the Healthy Side of Triathlon

Triathlon can be a wonderful, life-expanding experience. It can allow you to find meaning, satisfaction, and joy in an activity that promotes health, cultivates relationships, and extends your physical, psychological, and emotional horizons. It can create passion, bolster confidence, engender positive emotions, and encourage a life full of engagement, drive, and intensity. Yet for some, triathlon can be a harmful experience that is physically debilitating, emotionally crippling, and socially damaging. Because of the extreme nature of triathlon, in terms of the commitment needed, time and energy required, and physical demands involved, it can be a breeding ground and an outlet for unhealthy aspects of personality that can hurt self-esteem, promote obsessiveness, alienate family and friends, and lead to a life of anxiety, frustration, and unhappiness.

Triathlon attracts some of the healthiest people in the world who value fitness, competition, and the outdoors. It also draws some people who are not so psychologically healthy and who are looking to triathlon to fill a void in their lives. These people, rather than running (and biking and swimming) toward healthy goals, are trying to run (bike and swim) away from their problems and their demons. Which group you fall into depends on why you're involved in the sport, what you get out of your participation, and how it affects your life as a whole. One simple litmus test to determine whether you've gone to the "dark side" of triathlon is whether the sport hurts your physical health, relationships, or emotional well-being. Are you usually tired, sick, or injured? Have your family, friends, partners, and work relationships suffered? Are you more angst-ridden, irritable, and unhappy than not? This chapter is devoted to educating you about the dark side of triathlon and ensuring that you stay on the healthy side of the sport.

ENTERING THE DARK SIDE

People who enter the dark side of triathlon are driven by a variety of unhealthy motivations, including self-doubt, insecurity, and fear. At the center of these motivations is the need to feel better about themselves, safe and free from anxiety. By achieving triathlon success, those on the dark side believe they'll receive the respect and admiration they want from others, the love and value they crave from themselves, and the inner peace they are seeking. Unfortunately, these unhealthy needs can be exacerbated rather than alleviated by their involvement in triathlon.

Three concerns lie at the heart of why people go to the dark side of triathlon. Foremost is low self-esteem, in which people view themselves as lacking in competence and unworthy of love and respect from others and themselves. They get involved in triathlon in an attempt to show how capable they are and how deserving they are of love and respect. These triathletes approach the sport from a position of weakness in which they *need* to be successful to feel good about themselves. Unfortunately, because their needs are so great and their expectations are so extreme, participation in triathlon rarely satisfies that need.

People are also drawn to the dark side of triathlon by becoming overly invested in the sport. Their self-identity becomes excessively connected to their triathlon efforts. Ideally, triathlon should be just one small slice of the pie that is their self-identity, which should also include work, family, friends, and other interests and avocations. But when triathlon becomes the dominant slice of the pie, they may draw most of their beliefs and feelings about themselves from their triathlon pursuits. The unfortunate side to this over identification is that when things aren't going well in triathlon, such as when they experience overtraining, poor results, or injury, they feel negative about themselves, as if a part of themselves—that slice—has been removed.

Perfectionists are another group who are drawn to triathlon. Triathlon is the perfect sport for perfectionists. Because of its complexity, intensity, minute details, precise organization, and result orientation, the sport satisfies the punctilious needs of those whose standards are higher than high. Perfectionists are drawn to triathlon because it allows them to focus on the smallest details, gives them the sense of control that they crave, and creates an artificial world with the precise structure with which they are most comfortable.

Triathlon can also be the bane of perfectionists. They can start with a "perfect" world comprised of organized training, immaculately prepared equipment, detailed lists, and a structured routine, but the real world of triathlon is quite messy. Filled with unpredictable weather, equipment failures, and nutritional crises, triathlon is the antithesis of the perfect sport. A race day that begins superbly planned, highly organized, and well structured can quickly morph into a chaotic experience of perseverance in the face of unexpected adversity, improvisation in response to unplanned problems, and the need for flexibility in a constantly changing environment. What starts as a dream day for perfectionists can turn into a nightmare of frustration, lost control, and inflexibility.

Perfectionists have attached their self-esteem to their achievements, which, no matter how lofty they might be, are never enough to meet the unrealistic standards they have set for themselves. Perfectionists direct their often maniacal efforts to achieve the impossible goal of perfection in pursuit of feelings of competence and a happiness and contentment that they so desperately crave.

Triathletes who have gone to the dark side maintain their efforts despite their lack of success at finding what they want. These people tend to believe that they simply haven't done enough to achieve their goals rather than recognizing that their goals are misplaced. They are also loath to admit defeat in pursuit of their goals because such an admission would only confirm that they are failures unworthy of love and respect. Their intense and continuing triathlon efforts act as an anesthetic against the painful sense of inadequacy they feel in their lives. When they're training hard and feeling physical pain, they're distracted from the emotional pain that exists in their lives. Also, when they have small successes in training and races, they experience "highs" that, however briefly, offer them a respite from their angst.

The most unfortunate aspect of the dark side of triathlon is that all of the efforts that these people put into the sport are ultimately self-defeating. They put so much time and energy into their triathlon efforts in the belief that they will find what they are seeking, that they don't realize that they're looking for the wrong things in the wrong places. Not only are they not finding what they want, but they are kept from finding a new direction in which they can find what they're searching for.

Dangers of the Dark Side

Living on the dark side of triathlon isn't just a frustrating experience in which you never seem to find what you seek; it also presents a number of very real dangers that can be harmful. The most common danger of this unhealthy side of triathlon is overtraining. Because triathletes are driven to train and race, they tend to believe in the "more is better" approach to training that we referred to earlier, making them vulnerable to overtraining.

Illegal supplements are another physical danger for those who fall to the dark side. Triathlon is a supplement-intensive sport in which participants are encouraged to use a wide variety of specialized pills, drinks, and foods, all of which promise enhanced performance. Though all triathletes who want to perform at a higher level can be reasonably expected to take advantage of these nutritional tools, those who go to the dark side may be tempted to go beyond accepted and lawful supplements, and use illegal substances, for example, steroids and EPO (erythropoietin), to improve their performances. The use of illegal substances can be especially tempting as triathletes pursue coveted prizes, such as Hawaii Ironman® qualifying slots and USA triathlon international team selection, and, among pros, monetary incentives. Nina Kraft's disqualification due to a positive drug test after winning the 2004 Ironman® World Championships exemplifies the pressures that triathletes can feel that can lure them to the dark side.

The specter of other forms of cheating to gain a competitive advantage rises dramatically on the dark side. Perhaps the most notable type of cheating that we see in response to the siren's call of Hawaii Ironman® slots is drafting during the bike leg of qualifying races. Though clearly against the rules and associated with appropriate sanctions, drafting is a common sight in races where triathletes who have gone to the dark side are competing and where there is some tangible benefit to cheating.

The dangers of the dark side are not just physical in nature. Triathletes who live on the dark side put the sport as their highest priority and, as a result, may cause their relationships with family and friends to suffer from neglect. The desperate commitment that triathletes who are on the dark side make to the sport can cause them to lessen their commitment to their professional lives, either by taking work that is less demanding or financially rewarding or not devoting sufficient time to it. Finally, the greatest danger is the price that is paid in unhappiness. Despite all of the efforts of triathletes who are on the dark side to find peace and contentment, these efforts are usually counterproductive. Without exploring issues that led to the dark side, such as low self-esteem, narrow self-identity, and perfectionism, and choosing to leave the dark side, happiness is a largely unattainable goal.

I had cracked mentally and gave up, burned out—needed a break from the sport. I definitely lost my focus the past two years, and the results have shown it. I took a big break this spring, and I'm looking forward to getting going again.

—Peter Reid

Warning Signs of the Dark Side

You may now be asking yourself which side of triathlon you're on. Few triathletes would readily admit that they do triathlons for the wrong reasons. Still fewer may even be aware that they are on the dark side. We offer a number of warning signs you can look for in yourself to help you understand your relationship with triathlon.

The strongest indication of the dark side is a profound *need* to train that is expressed as a compulsion to work out with a frequency, intensity, and volume that is excessive and unbalanced. If you're on the dark side, you train anaerobically too much, swimming, biking, and running well beyond a reasonable threshold, often trying to keep up with faster triathletes. You may also have difficulty taking rest days during training weeks and recovery time after a high-intensity, high-volume training period. Tapering for a race is absolute torture for you, and you don't allow yourself adequate time to recover after races, feeling the need to get back to hard training for fear that you'll lose your fitness.

This need to train also manifests itself in the choices you make about how triathlon fits into your overall life. Because not training isn't an option, you may devote an inordinate amount of time to training at the expense of other parts of your life. As we have discussed several times throughout this book, relationships, work, and other interests and activities may suffer.

There are several psychological warning signs you can look for. Some pre-race nerves are normal, but if you experience significant performance anxiety in the days leading up to the race and just before the start, the dark side may be dictating your reactions. Your anxiety may be a response to a perceived threat in which how you perform in the race will affect how you feel about yourself as a person. The dark side causes every situation, whether training or a race, in which you could compare yourself to others, to be a potential threat to your self-esteem.

Excessive self-criticism is another warning sign of the dark side. When you struggle or perform poorly in some part of your training or you have a bad race, you castigate yourself beyond what is reasonable. You may dwell on it for days and have trouble letting go of your criticisms of yourself. Others may see your efforts and performances as perfectly adequate, but you hold yourself to an unfairly high standard. When you have a good workout or perform well in a race, you don't balance your criticism of your perceived failures with appropriate praise for your successes, and you find minute details of which to be critical.

Triathletes who have gone to the dark side often get in their own way. They engage in what is called self-defeating behavior, in which they do things that, on the surface, make them appear to be committed and hardworking, but in reality keep them from achieving their goals. They may, for example, train so hard that they become sick or injured, keeping them from racing up to their fullest ability. Their peers would express admiration at these efforts, thereby providing affirmation in the face of failure. This strategy protects their self-esteem without having to risk the possibility of real failure.

The presence of certain emotions is also a warning sign of being on the dark side. If you feel anxious, frustrated, depressed, or angry on a regular basis related to your triathlon, you may be living on the dark side. If the preponderance of emotions that you feel from triathlon is negative, take that as a red flag.

EIGHT KEYS TO TRIATHLON BALANCE

To ensure that you don't enter the dark side of triathlon (or that you get out of the dark side), keep the role that triathlon plays in your life in perspective and maintain a healthy balance of your involvement in the sport with your overall life. Triathlon should add to rather than detract from your life as a whole and should foster qualities and experiences that enhance other parts of your life, including your relationships, work, and other activities. Triathlon should contribute to your growth as a person, promoting admirable qualities, such as humility, passion, and patience. Triathlon should also discourage less desirable attributes, such as selfishness, perfectionism, and self-doubt. In other words, triathlon should make you a better person.

Be a human being, not a human doing. In our achievement-oriented, "it's all about results" world, many people can base how they feel about themselves on what they accomplish rather than who they are. Though being a "human doing" encourages people to work hard and achieve great success, there is rarely much joy in the accomplishments. Most of human doings' efforts are directed toward accomplishing goals and succeeding so they can validate their self-esteem and gain some modicum of peace. But they never feel any lasting contentment because human doings only briefly feel as good as their last accomplishment and are then dependent on their next achievement to continue to feel valued.

Human beings, in contrast, base how they feel about themselves on who they are as people—the values they hold, the way they treat others, the responsible way in which they behave. Are they kind, thoughtful, and compassionate? Do they work hard, have patience, and persist in the face of adversity? Being a human being doesn't mean that you will lose interest in achieving and being successful. To the contrary, it liberates you from the fear of achieving because success and failure are no longer so centrally connected to your self-esteem. The removal of this threat to your self-esteem allows you to pursue success from a position of strength in which you want to seek out challenges, take risks, and fully realize your ability. It also allows you to accept the inevitable failures you will experience in pursuit of your goals. There is no pressure—from you or others—that interferes with human beings becoming successful. Human beings connect their passions and commitment to their efforts so what results is both success and tremendous satisfaction and joy in those efforts.

Redefine success and failure. Our culture has defined success and failure in a way that is narrow, limiting, and that ultimately will interfere with your achieving success and avoiding failure. Success has been defined simplistically in terms of results and winning. The message is that you must win to be valued. If you don't win, then your performance is insignificant. Buying into this definition for your triathlon participation makes success largely unattainable. At the same time, our culture has made failure even more intolerable to contemplate—not living up to our culture's definition of success makes you a failure.

Blindly having accepted society's narrow definitions of success and failure takes away your power to decide how you wish to define them. By buying into these limiting definitions of success and failure rather than choosing definitions based on your own values, you're forced down a path that is, for most people, impossible to attain and that was not truly yours.

For triathlon to be a truly meaningful and rewarding experience, create your own interpretations of success and failure. Broaden your definition of success to include expending great effort in pursuit of your goals, gaining satisfaction and joy in your training, having fun at races no matter what your result, staying focused on the process of each race, achieving personal bests, or contributing to the sport through triathlon club involvement and volunteering.

> *My mistakes, failures, injuries, illnesses, and setbacks ... have allowed me to take myself to the physical, mental, and emotional edge. My simple philosophy is that success comes from picking yourself up from your mistakes. Failures are only failures if you don't learn from them and turn them into future successes.*
>
> —Jackie Gallagher,
> 1996 ITU world champion

Whereas we broaden our definition of success, we narrow our definition of failure. Instead of an unhealthy definition of failure that could include failing to win, disappointing others, not being perfect, feeling incompetent, and not being worthy of love and respect, we limit failure to not giving your best effort and not enjoying the experience. This definition of failure is entirely within your control and doesn't carry the emotional baggage of the more commonly believed definition of failure. In this narrower context, your reaction to poor performance is one of disappointment, but you still enjoy the experience, letting it go and using the lessons learned from failure to become more successful in the future.

Keep triathlon in perspective. Triathlon is an absorbing sport. You can become so involved with its many facets, from training to nutrition to gear to triathlon club activities to races, that, without realizing it, it can take over your life. If it gains dominance over you and you begin to set all your priorities and make all your decisions based on triathlon, your overall life may suffer. Beyond the time commitment and practical involvement, the real danger is that you may become overly connected to triathlon and, as we have discussed, invest too much of your self-esteem in your participation. When this happens, you can lose perspective on the role that the sport plays in your life and you can be drawn to the dark side.

The ability to maintain perspective on how triathlon fits into your life will not only affect your training and race efforts, but also essential aspects of your overall life. What is most critical is that you realize that triathlon can be an important part of your life, but it is not life itself. With this view of the sport, it can still play a central role for you and be a wonderful source of satisfaction and enjoyment, but it won't become a burden to your triathlon efforts or other parts of your life.

Each year the pressure from sponsors and other people would become greater. Each year I would have to reflect again and again on my ultimate goals for being out there; I'd say, "The reason why I exercise is because I like the game and I like being healthy." This would remind me to stick with my goals and be consistent.

—Dave Scott

Maintain balance. Triathlon can be a sport that breeds imbalance. Because of its complexity and the time and energy that are required, it's challenging to maintain life balance while being committed to the sport. Yet balance is essential to leading a meaningful, satisfying, and joyful life. Balance means keeping triathlon in a healthy place in your life and maintaining respect for all parts of your life. You can devote sufficient time to achieve your triathlon goals. You have time to share with family and friends. You're able to remain fully committed to your professional life. And you can spend time enjoying other activities that you value. Balance doesn't just refer to a particular day, week, or month. It could also mean over the course of a year in which you tip the scale of your life's balance toward triathlon for six months and then you tip it back to other parts of your life the remainder of the year.

Maintaining balance is particularly difficult when you're training for a longer-distance race, such as an Ironman. The inordinate amount of time and energy that's necessary to prepare for long races largely precludes having true balance. But maintaining some semblance of balance, what we call "balance within the imbalance," is still a worthy goal. Balance within the imbalance involves finding small opportunities to infuse balance into your otherwise lopsided life. For example, commit one full afternoon on weekends after training to spend with your family, spend one evening a week doing extra work that you might have neglected because of your shortened hours at work, or catch an early dinner and a movie on Friday night and still be in bed early enough to get a good night's sleep in preparation for Saturday's long ride.

Some would say that if triathlons aren't first priority, you can't be best, but ... life is about balance. I wouldn't do my best if my priorities weren't straight.

—Barb Lindquist,
2004 U.S. Olympic Triathlon Team

Have healthy expectations. Living in a result-oriented culture, we tend to create expectations for ourselves based on our results. A great lesson you may have learned from triathlon is that you can't always control your race results. You can give a great effort, but because of a variety of factors outside of your control, for example, the weather, course conditions, or mechanical problems, you may not achieve the results that you had hoped for. If you believe our culture, then you will have to judge yourself as having failed.

Having healthy expectations means setting goals over which you have control and that you can achieve if you give your best effort. Healthy expectations can involve being completely prepared to have a successful race or enjoying your race experience. They can mean responding well to adversity or persisting when you're really hurting. The key is to establish expectations over which you have control and that will encourage success (as you define it) and satisfaction in their pursuit.

Strive for excellence, not perfection. We've already emphasized how unhealthy the pursuit of perfection is and how it will lead to neither success nor happiness. Because of the unpredictable nature of triathlon, we suggest that perfection is a goal that is both unattainable and undesirable. Our antidote to perfection is excellence, which we define as doing your best most of the time while accepting that things will go wrong and using the mistakes as learning experiences. Excellence takes the positive qualities of perfection, for example, setting high standards and working hard to achieve goals, and rejects its unhealthy aspects, such as failure being unacceptable and criticizing oneself for not living up to impossibly high standards. Excellence means giving your best effort on any given day, allowing that problems may arise, and adapting to the changing situations in a positive way. Excellence relieves you of the burden of everything having to be perfect, encourages the pursuit of your goals as challenges rather than threats, and enables you to remain positive and calm as you constructively deal with the unexpected tests that triathlon throws at you.

Feel the love and joy. Triathlon should be about love: love of yourself, love of the sport, and love for others. Yet because triathlon is a competitive sport, it can sometimes turn into a love for results: times, placings, and rankings. If you become overly focused on the results, you may lose your true love of triathlon. Without that passion for all things triathlon, you may find that, in time, your interest and motivation to train and race may wane.

One of my issues [racing pro] was one of expectations. What others expected. When you race at that level for that long you start to think that's all you are and what you are. One race I realized that no one really cared. Not one spectator, not one peer, sponsors. It's not going to have an impact on their day in how you solely do in one race. I learned to just go out and give it my best shot on the day. Just go out and do it.

—Paul Huddle

Love the process of triathlon—turning laps in the pool, pedal strokes on the bike, and strides on a run.

Love the experience and you'll get the results you want even though you aren't focused on them. If you love training, you're going to put in the time necessary to gain the fitness you need to achieve your goals. At races, because you're unconcerned with your results, you'll be more confident, relaxed, and focused, less anxious about how you'll perform and better able to perform up to your ability. The true end result is that you have a wonderful triathlon experience and you often get the results you want.

Tremendous joy can be found in the triathlon experience. Enjoy giving your best effort, improving your swimming, biking, and running, reveling in the heat of competition, and getting to know like-minded people. Triathlon remains a joy when it acts as an antidote for stress and a healthy escape from the demands of your life. It continues to be joyful when you maintain a positive balance of physical exertion and rest, and your time commitment to triathlon doesn't cause you to sacrifice other parts of your life. Triathlon is a joy when you're excited about and look forward to training, and races are fun and stimulating. You can also find joy by surrounding yourself with other triathletes who get joy from the sport. Enjoy the outdoors, meet the ongoing challenges, and savor the feeling you have after a great workout. Find joy in the changes you see in your body and mind. Staying continually connected to those feelings is the surest way to gain the maximum enjoyment out of triathlon.

Appreciate the benefits. Triathlon offers you many physical, mental, social, and spiritual benefits. It encourages exercise, good nutrition, and a healthy lifestyle. Cross training provides you with a level of balanced fitness—strength, endurance, flexibility—that may be unparalleled in sport. Triathlon gives you opportunities to increase your motivation, confidence, and focus, to relieve stress, learn about emotions, and develop discipline, patience, persistence, and perseverance. Triathlon introduces you to passionate, interesting, and committed people with positive attitudes who share common interests and goals, and who live spirited and vigorous lifestyles. Triathlon has a strong spiritual component; it challenges you to push your limits and expand your horizons. Triathlon presents you with opportunities that can teach essential life lessons to help you grow. The sport can be a source of profound meaning, satisfaction, and enjoyment. Whoever or whatever you worship spiritually, the benefits we just mentioned enable you to get closer to your faith and manifest it more fully in your life. Ultimately, triathlon offers you many and diverse experiences through which you can enhance the quality of your life.

My [triathlon] program is my little secret in the music business. It's so great to have a hobby that has nothing to do with my work. I am stronger physically, mentally, even emotionally as a result of the training. It has been a real self-esteem builder for me to realize at my age I can do something new and different that makes me feel good.

—Shawn Colvin, Grammy winner

TRIATHLETE SPOTLIGHT: TOM

Tom, age 37, grew up in a family where both of his parents were perfectionists who pushed him and his siblings to excel in every aspect of their lives. The high expectations that his parents set drove him to succeed in his professional life, but he paid a price for his achievements. He never felt he was good enough despite his efforts at perfection. He was obsessive about everything he committed to. Tom was terrified of failure and drove himself relentlessly to keep from failing. He never thought of himself as a happy person.

When he was introduced to triathlon, Tom knew he had found a sport that was made for him; its intensity, complexity, and demands fed right into his personality. He took meticulous care of his bike. In training, no workout was ever hard enough or long enough, and it was unthinkable for him to take time off to recover. No matter how well he did in races, he was never satisfied with his efforts or results. He developed a series of overuse injuries that he kept trying to train through, forcing him to stop training and racing all together. This void caused him to feel frustrated, angry, and depressed. At the urging of his girlfriend, he decided to see a sport psychologist, Dr. B., to help him find some solutions to what he was feeling.

It quickly became clear to Dr. B. that Tom's unforgiving personality was not only negatively influencing his triathlon efforts, but his overall happiness and well-being as well. He began to explore with Tom his perfectionism and how it affected his life. Tom, for the first time, started to see why he was so perfectionistic and how it interfered with his triathlon pursuits and caused his general unhappiness. With these realizations, he was committed to making changes.

Over time, Tom's perspectives on triathlon (and life) were transformed. With Dr. B.'s help, he altered his definitions of success and failure, placing greater emphasis on finding satisfaction in his efforts rather than just his results and recognizing that some failure was necessary to achieve success. He created healthier expectations that focused on his efforts, progress, and enjoyment in doing triathlons. His biggest challenge was letting go of his perfectionism because it was so closely tied to his self-esteem. With help from his girlfriend, he learned that he didn't have to be perfect to be loved and respected; he could fail periodically and still be a good person.

(continued on next page)

(continued from previous page)

Dr. B. helped Tom focus on the wonderful benefits of triathlon—physical health, psychological and emotional well-being, friendships—and how the sport enhanced his life. Most importantly, Tom connected for the first time with the love he had for triathlon and the joy that the sport brought him, not the extreme effort or the results, but rather the simple acts of swimming, biking, and running. For the first time in his life, he felt a weight lifted off his shoulders, and he believed that not only could he freely pursue healthy goals in triathlon, but he could also find happiness in life.

Afterword

To be motivated, confident, intense, and focused. To be an emotional master. To endure and overcome physical challenges. To be your best ally. To perform your best consistently under the most demanding conditions. These are the skills that Prime Triathlon can help you develop.

Why is Prime Triathlon so important to you that you would read this book and put such time and effort into triathlon? Your answer is a personal one. For some, it may be to have more fun in the sport. For others, it may be to become the best triathlete they possibly can. For still others, it may be to have better results.

We would like to believe, though, that the most compelling reason why you want to achieve Prime Triathlon is to master the *mental race*, what we described in the introduction as the most important and difficult race in which you compete. If you can remove the obstacles that keep you from performing your best, you clear the path to fulfillment of your goals in triathlon and meaning in your efforts. More importantly though, by succeeding at the mental race, you open the door to living your most meaningful, satisfying, and joyful life. We hope that as you have read *The Triathlete's Guide to Mental Training*, you've thought, "Hey, this could apply to my work" or "This relates to my relationships." Because triathlon, like life, is filled with challenges, struggles, excitement, setbacks, failures, and ultimately, success—and to triumph in the mental race is to seize victory in life itself.

JIM TAYLOR, PH.D.
TERRI SCHNEIDER

References

Apter, M. J. (1989). *Reversal theory: Motivation, emotion, and personality.* London: Routledge.

Budgett, R. (1990). Overtraining syndrome. *British Journal of Sports Medicine, 24,* 231-236.

Budgett, R. (1994). The overtraining syndrome. *British Medical Journal, 309,* 465-468.

Butler, R. J., & Hardy, L. (1992). The performance profile: Theory and application. *The Sport Psychologist, 6,* 253-264.

Cannon, W. B. (1932). *The Wisdom of the Body.* New York: Norton.

Cautela, J. R., & Wisocki, P. A. (1977). Thought-stoppage procedure: Description, application, and learning theory applications. *Psychological Records, 27,* 255-264.

Conroy, D. E. (2001). Fear of failure: An exemplar for social development research in sport. *Quest, 53,* 165-183.

Conroy, D. E., Poczwardowski, A., & Henschen, K. P. (2001). Evaluative criteria and consequences associated with failure and success for elite athletes and performing artists. *Journal of Applied Sport Psychology, 13,* 300-322.

Druckman, D., & Bjork, R. A. (1991). *In the mind's eye: Enhancing human performance.* Washington, DC: National Academy Press.

Ericsson, K., & Charnes, N. (1994). Expert performance: Its structure and acquisition. *American Psychologist, 49,* 725-747.

Foster, C., & Lehmann, M. (1999). Overtraining syndrome. *Insider, 7,* 1-6.

Froehlich, J. (1993). Overtraining syndrome. In J. Heil (Ed.), *Psychology of sport injury* (pp. 59-70). Champaign, IL: Human Kinetics.

Fry, R. W., Morton, A. R., & Keast, D. (1992a). Overtraining syndrome and the chronic fatigue syndrome, Part 1. *New Zealand Journal of Sports Medicine, 19,* 48-52.

Fry, R. W., Morton, A. R., & Keast, D. (1992b). Periodization of training stress—A Review. *Canadian Journal of Sports Science, 17,* 234-240.

Hanin, Y. L. (1999). Individual zones of optimal functioning (IZOF) model: Emotions-performance relationships in sport. In Y. L. Hanin (Ed.), *Emotions in sport* (pp. 65–89). Champaign, IL: Human Kinetics.

Hawley, C. J., & Schoene, R. B. (2003). Overtraining: Why training too hard, too long, doesn't work. *The Physician and Sports Medicine, 31*, 16–33.

Heil, J. (1993). *Psychology of sport injury.* Champaign, IL: Human Kinetics.

Henschen, K. P. (2001). Athletic staleness and burnout: Diagnosis, prevention, and treatment. In J. M. Williams (Ed.), *Applied sport psychology: Personal growth to peak performance* (pp. 445–455). Mountain View, CA: Mayfield.

Ievleva, L., & Orlick, T. (1991). Mental links to enhancing healing: An exploratory study. *The Sport Psychologist, 5*, 25–40.

Jacobson, E. (1930). *Progressive relaxation.* Chicago: University of Chicago Press.

Johnson, R. J. (June 9, 2000). Overtraining 101: How to overtrain. Retrieved from http://www.letsrun.com/overtrain.html

Keast, D., & Morton, A. R. (May 1, 2002). Overtraining. Retrieved from http://www.sportsci.org/encyc/drafts/Overtraining.doc

Kentta, G., & Hassmen, P. (1998). Overtraining and recovery: A conceptual model. *Sports Medicine, 26*, 25–39.

Kuipers, H., & Keizer, H. A. (1988). Overtraining in elite athletes: Review and directions for the future. *Sports Medicine, 6*, 79–92.

Martin, A. J., & Marsh, H. W. (2003). Fear of failure: Friend or foe? *Australian Psychologist, 38*, 31–38.

Moran, A. (1996). *The psychology of concentration in sport performers: A cognitive analysis.* East Sussex, UK: Psychology.

Nideffer, R. M. (1981). *The ethics and practice of applied sport psychology.* Ithaca, NY: Mouvement.

Raglin, J. S., & Hanin, Y. L. (1999). Competitive anxiety. In Y. L. Hanin (Ed.), *Emotions in sport* (pp. 93–111). Champaign, IL: Human Kinetics.

Schmidt, R. A., & Wrisberg, C. A. (2000). *Motor learning and performance* (2nd ed.). Champaign, IL: Human Kinetics.

Seligman, M. E. P. (1998). *Learned helplessness: How to change your mind and your life.* New York: Free Press.

Silva, J. (1990). An analysis of the training stress syndrome in competitive athletics. *Journal of Applied Sport Psychology, 2*, 5-20.

Singer, R. N., Murphey, M., & Tennant, L. K. (Eds.) (1993). *Handbook of research on sport psychology*. New York: MacMillan.

Sonstroem, R. J. (1984). An overview of anxiety in sport. In J. M. Silva III & R. S. Weinberg (Eds.), *Psychological foundations of sport* (pp. 104-117). Champaign, IL: Human Kinetics.

Taylor, J. (2001). *Prime sport: Triumph of the athlete mind*. New York: iUniverse.

Taylor, J. (November 2002). Pain is your friend. *Inside Triathlon*, pp. 54-55.

Taylor, J., & Cusimano, K. (October 8, 2003). Mental training for endurance athletes. Continuing education workshop presented at the annual meetings of the Association for the Advancement of Applied Sport Psychology, Philadelphia, PA.

Taylor, J., & Taylor, S. (1997). *Psychological approaches to sports injury rehabilitation*. Gaithersburg, MD: Aspen.

Taylor, J., & Wilson, G. S. (2002). Intensity regulation and sport performance. In J. L. Van Raalte & B. W. Brewer (Eds.), *Exploring sport and exercise psychology* (pp. 99-130). Washington, DC: APA.

Taylor, J., Stone, K. R., Mullin, M. J., Ellenbecker, T., & Walgenbach, A. (2003). *Comprehensive sports injury management*. Austin, TX: Pro-ed.

Van Raalte, J. L., & Brewer, B. W. (Eds.) (1996). *Exploring sport and exercise psychology*. Washington, DC: APA.

Weinberg, R. S., & Gould, D. (2003). *Foundations of sport and exercise psychology* (3rd ed). Champaign, IL: Human Kinetics.

Williams, J. M. (Ed.) (1998). *Applied sport psychology: Personal growth to peak performance* (3rd ed.) (pp. 219-236). Palo Alto, CA: Mayfield.

Williams, J. M., & Harris, D. V. (2001). Relaxation and energizing techniques for regulation of arousal. In J. M. Williams (Ed.), *Applied sport psychology: Personal growth to peak performance* (pp. 229-246). Mountain View, CA: Mayfield.

Index

About the Authors

Jim Taylor, Ph.D.

Jim is internationally recognized for his work in the psychology of endurance sport. Jim has been a consultant to USA Triathlon and works with world-class and age-group endurance athletes in cycling, running, triathlon, and swimming. A former alpine ski racer who competed internationally, Jim is a second-degree black belt in karate, a sub-three-hour marathoner, and an Ironman triathlete. Jim is the author of ten books, including the *Prime Sport* book series, *Psychological Approaches to Sports Injury Rehabilitation*, and *Comprehensive Sports Injury Management*. He has published over 400 articles and has given more than 500 workshops and presentations throughout North America and Europe. To learn more, visit www.drjimtaylor.com.

Terri Schneider

Terri is a former professional triathlete and one of the top female multi-sport endurance athletes in the world. Terri has competed internationally in seven Eco-Challenge Expedition races, the Mild Seven Outdoor Quest in China, the ESPN X Games Adventure Race, the Raid Gauloises, twenty-two Ironman triathlons, and many ultrarunning events. She is a frequent speaker to athletic and corporate groups, as well as a regular contributor to various sport- and health-related magazines and websites. She has coached triathletes, adventure racers, runners, cyclists, and swimmers for fifteen years. To learn more, visit www.terrischneider.com.